ACUPRESSURE
MADE
SIMPLE

Also by Deborah Bleecker

Virus Remedies Guidebook
Acupuncture Points Handbook
Natural Back Pain Solutions
Acupuncture Points Quick Guide
Shingles Relief
Acupuncture for Migraines
Insomnia Relief

ACUPRESSURE
MADE
SIMPLE

Easily Treat Yourself
for
Common Ailments

Deborah Bleecker, LAc, MSOM

Disclaimer

This book contains the opinions and ideas of the author. It is intended to provide helpful and informative material on the subjects addressed. It is sold with the understanding that the author and publisher are not engaged in rendering medical, health, psychological or any other type of advice or services in the book. If the reader needs personal, medical, health, or other assistance or advice, a competent professional should be consulted.

Care has been taken to confirm the accuracy of the information presented and to describe generally accepted practices. However, the authors, editors, and publisher are not responsible for errors or omissions or for any consequences from application of the information in this book and make no warranty, express or implied, with respect to the contents of the publication.

The author and publisher disclaim any responsibility for any liability, loss or risk, either personal or otherwise that occurs as a consequence, directly or indirectly, of the use and application of the contents of this book.

Contents

Introduction

Acupressure is a safe and effective way to treat yourself for many ailments. Since there are over 1,000 recorded acupuncture points, how do you choose which one will work best? That is what this book is about. As a licensed acupuncturist, I have been teaching my patients acupressure to help them treat themselves for over 20 years.

My goal with this book is to make acupressure easy to understand and use effectively. I have chosen the most effective acupressure points, and they are explained in a way that makes sense to a layperson.

In most cases, there are only a few points you need to use for each ailment. That is because acupuncture points are so strong, and so effective, that you might only need to know the *one* point that will work best. There is no reason to use five points, when one will do. I explain which point to try first for each ailment.

I have a Master of Science degree in Oriental Medicine. This is the standard three year graduate level program in Chinese medicine that licensed acupuncturists in America complete. In this program we spend an entire year learning how to locate and treat over 400 acupuncture points. We also learn how to combine the points to treat disease.

Since I have been treating patients over 20 years, I have also studied health supplements extensively. Although this book focuses on acupressure, I could not leave out treatment notes for supplements that I recommend to my patients to help them heal faster. These are the most dependable and highest quality supplements. I am not compensated by or affiliated with these companies in any way, but I have found them to be very effective, and it will save you some time and money to buy the most effective supplements.

Acupuncture points regulate the body's function. Your body knows what healthy is. It is in your DNA. You just have to help it to regulate itself and restore healthy function.

Acupuncture points relieve pain by restoring healthy circulation. Your body can heal itself when there is good circulation.

Top Ten Acupressure Points

Although every acupuncturist has favorite points, the points below are the most commonly used in many acupuncture clinics. The reason they are so popular is that they are very strong, and they have many functions.

The information below is a small excerpt of my book, *Acupuncture Points Handbook*. I have chosen the most commonly used indications of the points, to make it simple to understand and use the points.

In alphabetical order, my choice for the top ten points:

Heart 7
Kidney 3
Kidney 6
Kidney 7
Large Intestine 4
Large Intestine 11
Liver 3
Pericardium 6
Spleen 6
Stomach 36

A cun is about the width of your thumb knuckle. This will be explained in detail later.

Heart 7

Located at the wrist crease, on the radial side of the flexor *carpi ulnaris* tendon. You might have two or three of these creases, but this point is located at the level of the largest wrist crease. If you wiggle your little finger, you will feel the tendon move.

Heart 7

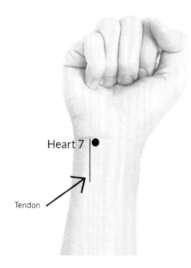

Functions and Common Usage

Heart 7 is used for anxiety, it calms the mind, treats arrhythmias, palpitations, insomnia, and irritability.

Kidney 3

Located in the depression between the inner ankle bone, and the back of the leg. Locate the point halfway between the tip of the inner ankle bone and the back of the leg.

Kidney 3

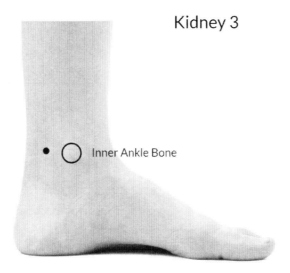

Inner Ankle Bone

Functions and Common Usage

Kidney 3 is the most important and most commonly used point on the Kidney meridian. It treats asthma, deafness from kidney weakness, heel pain, incontinence, insomnia, urination issues, tinnitus, and urgent urination.

Kidney 6

Located one cun below the inner ankle bone.

Kidney 6

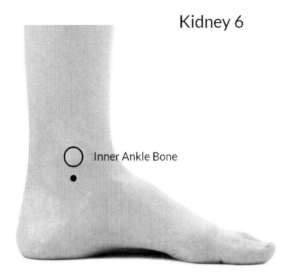

Inner Ankle Bone

Functions and Common Usage
Kidney 6 calms the mind, treats weak urination, edema, frequent urination, hot flashes, insomnia, uterine prolapse, and strengthens the kidneys.

Kidney 7
Located 2 cun on a direct line above Kidney 3.

Functions and Common Usage
Kidney 7 treats lower back pain, nephritis, foot pain, incontinence, edema, frequent urination, and it regulates the bladder.

Kidney 7

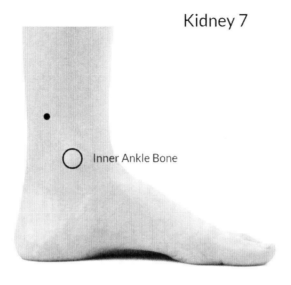

Inner Ankle Bone

Large Intestine 4
Located between the first and second hand bones, in the middle of the second hand bone, on the thumb side. This point should not be used by pregnant women, because it could induce labor.

Large Intestine 4

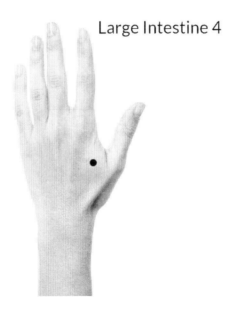

Functions and Common Usage
Large Intestine 4 treats allergies, arm pain, cold and flu, hand pain, headaches, hives, induces labor, regulates the immune system, sinus congestion, and nosebleed. It treats the eyes, nose, mouth, and ears. It is famous for treating headaches.

Large Intestine 11
Located halfway between the elbow crease and the elbow. Locate with the arm bent, as shown in the image. It is easy to use your own thumb to treat this point.

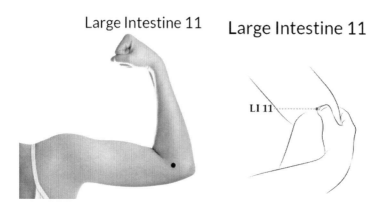

Large Intestine 11   Large Intestine 11

LI 11

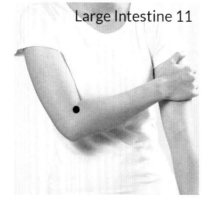

Large Intestine 11

Functions and Common Usage

Large Intestine 11 treats allergies, arm atrophy, arm pain, elbow pain, high blood pressure, constipation, hives, itching, rashes, shoulder pain and stiffness, skin diseases, and it strengthens the immune system.

Liver 3

Located between the first and second toes, about 1.5 cun above the web of the toe. Please note that the size of your feet bones determines how far this point is from the toe web, everyone is different. It is located in the depression between the first and second feet bones.

To locate Liver 3 you can run your finger along the toe web to the foot bones, you will find a small indentation right before you get to the bones of the feet. The image shows the point with a circle around it, so you can see that Liver 3 is located in a small hollow on the foot.

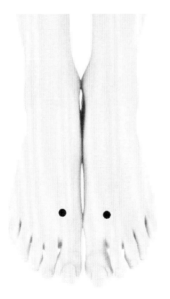

Liver 3

Liver 3

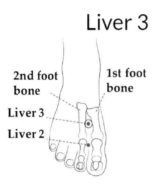

Functions and Common Usage

Liver 3 treats stress, dizziness, eye conditions, irregular menstruation, high blood pressure, insomnia, nausea, vertigo, and depression.

Pericardium 6

Located 2 cun above the wrist crease, between the tendons in the middle of the forearm.

Pericardium 6

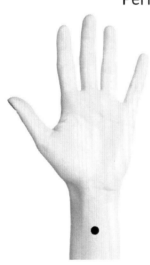

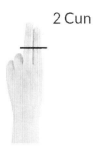

2 Cun

Functions and Common Usage
Pericardium 6 treats anxiety, calms the stomach, treats
hiccups, insomnia, palpitations, regulates the heart, and
treats nausea.

Spleen 6
Located on the inside of the leg, 3 cun above the tip of the
inner ankle bone, behind the shin bone. Locate with your
whole hand on the tip of the ankle bone. You can easily locate
the point by pressing on the area to find the back border of
the bone.

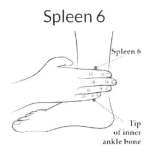

Spleen 6

Spleen 6

Tip
of inner
ankle bone

Spleen 6

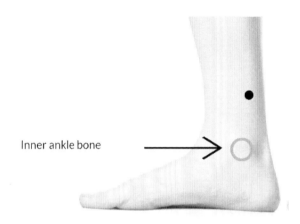

Inner ankle bone

Functions and Common Usage
Spleen 6 treats anemia, anxiety, hormonal imbalances, foot paralysis, headache, edema or water retention, high blood pressure, infertility, insomnia, labor induction, stress, and uterine prolapse.

Stomach 36
Located 3 cun below the eye of the knee, and one finger width from the front edge of the shin bone.

Stomach 36 can be located several ways. You can place your hand over your knee to measure the point. The index finger is placed at the level of the eyes of the knee, which are the small depressions on both sides of your kneecap. The point is just below your little finger. You can also cross reference the location by using the tibia, or shin bone.

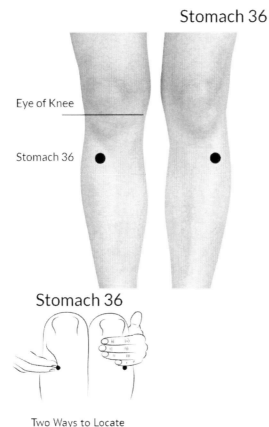

Stomach 36

Eye of Knee

Stomach 36

Stomach 36

Two Ways to Locate

Functions and Common Usage

Stomach 36 is perhaps the most commonly used point in acupuncture. It is easiest to understand the many functions of the point by looking at the categories.

Regulates and strengthens the Spleen and Stomach

Treats belching, abdominal fullness, diarrhea, constipation, nausea, poor appetite, vomiting, diaphragm spasms, fatigue, and difficulty swallowing.

Regulates and strengthens the Lungs

Treats asthma, cough, and shortness of breath.

Regulates and moistens the intestines
Treats constipation and diarrhea, as well as intestinal abscess.

Regulates and strengthens the immune system
Treats allergies, colds, and flu, and hives.

In addition to the above, it treats knee pain, leg paralysis (see my section on stroke recovery), knee weakness, and high blood pressure.

Stomach 36 is one of the best points on the body to improve energy levels. It improves digestion, and relieves fatigue. It is called "Leg Three Miles," because the saying goes that even when you are at the point of exhaustion and cannot go on any longer, you can treat this point and walk three more miles.

Chinese Medicine Quick Guide

Although it is not necessary for you to understand Chinese medicine theory to use acupressure, I wanted to include a little information on this. I am including a very basic explanation to make this simple.

Chinese Medicine Diagnosis
A Chinese medicine diagnosis includes asking numerous questions. These questions tell us how your body is working. The questions might not seem to be related to your ailment, but they are in Chinese medicine. We will look at your tongue to see the general color and coating, as well as the shape. We take your pulse, which gives us more information about your health.

There are dozens of what we call *Organ Patterns* in Chinese medicine. You can have one, or you can have many of them. After a diagnosis has been made, acupuncture works to treat the underlying imbalances. Symptoms that seem to be unrelated to your health issue, can be very important in making your Chinese medicine diagnosis. The symptoms go away when the underlying imbalance is resolved.

Yin and Yang
You might have heard about Yin and Yang and wondered what they were. The theory behind them is pretty extensive, but I want you to have a basic idea of what they are, because certain acupuncture points treat the Yin, and some treat the Yang.

Think of Yang as hot, dry, and energy. It is related to the drive, and testosterone can be associated with it. As we age, our Kidneys decline. That causes a reduction in hormones. Yin is the cool, and moist. Yin correlates to estrogen.

Yin and Yang must be sufficient for the body to be healthy. There are many herbal tonics that are used in Chinese medicine to strengthen the Yin and Yang of the kidneys to improve health as you age.

Please remember that only *one* symptom is necessary to indicate that organ pattern is relevant for a health issue. In many cases, that is all someone will have, one symptom. These symptoms are combined with other factors such as the pulse and tongue for a complete picture. This is a starting point in diagnosis.

Kidney Organ Patterns

The most common imbalances in the Kidneys are a Yin or Yang deficiency. The kidneys are the root of your health in Chinese medicine theory. If you can keep your kidneys healthy, you will be less likely to get sick.

Kidney Yang Deficiency

Common symptoms of Kidney Yang deficiency include lower back pain, weak or painful knees, weak legs, feeling cold when others are comfortable, impotence, premature ejaculation, fatigue, frequent or profuse urination, apathy, swelling in the legs, and fertility problems.

Kidney Yin Deficiency

Common symptoms of a Kidney Yin deficiency are dizziness, tinnitus, poor memory, hearing issues or deafness, dry mouth at night, thirst, lower back pain, bone aches, insomnia, and night sweats. A Kidney Yin deficiency can be correlated to an estrogen deficiency.

Spleen and Stomach Organ Patterns

The Spleen in Chinese medicine theory is completely different from the function in Western medicine. The Spleen in Chinese medicine is associated with digestion and energy production. The most common imbalance is Spleen Qi deficiency.

Spleen Qi Deficiency

A weak Spleen can cause a lack of appetite, abdominal bloating after eating, fatigue, pale complexion, weak arms and legs, loose stools. A spleen weakness can also cause excess fluid to be retained in the body.

Heart Organ Patterns

The Heart is affected by all emotions. Heart imbalances often cause anxiety, and insomnia.

Heart Qi Deficiency

When the energy of the Heart is weak, it can cause heart palpitations, shortness of breath on exertion, unusual sweating, pale face, and fatigue. Palpitations are when you feel your heart beating.

Lung Organ Patterns

The Lungs can be treated with acupuncture to resolve colds and flu, treat asthma, bronchitis, and any ailment associated with the lungs. Strong lungs ensure healthy energy levels.

Lung Qi Deficiency

A Lung Qi deficiency means the lung function is weak, which can cause shortness of breath, coughing, a weak voice, and a dislike of speaking. This can also be a side effect of a cold or flu. The coughing during a cold weakens the Lungs, which can cause a chronic weak cough.

Liver Organ Patterns

The Liver in Chinese medicine theory is very different from the modern medicine theory. The Liver is affected by stress. Being stressed out regularly causes liver energy imbalances.

Liver Qi Stagnation

Liver Qi stagnation causes feeling irritated or stressed, sighing, hiccup, depression, nausea, vomiting, acid reflux, belching, difficulty swallowing, irregular periods, painful periods, breast distention, and lumps in the breast or under the arms.

Liver Fire

Liver Fire causes severe irritability, sudden outbursts of anger, tinnitus, and headaches on the side of the head, dizziness, thirst, bitter taste, and a sudden flushed feeling when angry. Liver 2 is the best point for Liver Fire.

Acupuncture during Pregnancy

There are points that are not to be used during pregnancy. You will find that different sources cite different points. The most commonly listed points to avoid during pregnancy are Spleen 6, Large Intestine 4, Ren 4, Bladder 31, 32, 33, 34, Gallbladder 21, and Bladder 60. These points are contraindicated during pregnancy, which means they should be avoided during pregnancy. If you are pregnant, please consult a licensed acupuncturist for help.

How to Make Acupressure Work for You

There is an expression in Chinese medicine called "Getting the Qi." This means that when a point is stimulated, whether by a needle, or your fingers, the point has to be activated. If you press for just a minute, the point is not likely to have been activated enough to have an effect.

Sensation of Qi
Acupressure does not give you the same type of sensations you get with acupuncture. The most likely sensation is a slight numbness if you have been working on the point a while. The sensations you could feel include itching, tingling, numbness, aching, and warmth.

When acupuncture is done, the needles are left in place for about 30 minutes. In some cases they are left in less time, but that is a common amount of time. When I treat patients, I leave the needles in a minimum of 20 minutes. If I am treating tight back muscles, I might leave the needles in a little longer, because that person might need a little longer for the muscles to relax. The normal physiological response to an acupuncture needle inserted into a tight muscle is for the muscle to relax after about 30 minutes.

The effect you get from acupuncture might take seconds, but you will notice that your body will continue to react as the day goes on, and the next day you might be significantly better. This is especially true when treating tight muscles. It takes a little time for the body to adjust to the treatment.

When doing acupressure, you need to press long enough to activate the point. In my experience, it is a minimum of five minutes. What I typically do is press on one side for five minutes, then switch to the other side. So I might start with Large Intestine 4 on the left hand, massage or press for five minutes, then treat the right hand for five minutes. With acupressure I would expect some results within an hour for things like allergies or constipation. If you are treating hormone or digestive issues, you might not see signs that it is working, but the results will be more obvious after a week.

Your reaction and rate of healing is determined by how many ailments your body has to heal, and how bad it is. If you have had a problem for 10 years, it will take longer than treating something you got that day, such as an allergic reaction. If your general health is pretty good, you will see results faster. Don't let that discourage you. You are starting now. You will continue to improve if you do not give up.

Treatment Frequency
In China, acupuncture is done daily, and a series of 10 treatments is considered a course of treatment. In hospitals in China treatment is done twice daily, and Chinese herbal medicine is prescribed. In the West, we tend to see patients twice weekly. If a patient is in a hurry to get better, we would treat more than twice a week to stabilize the person.

 In some cases, patients can get acupuncture only once a week. They still get better! It will take a little longer to resolve the root cause of their health problems, but they will continue to improve over time and there is no reason to not get acupuncture for your health problems if you cannot go as often as you want to. Your acupuncturist will work with you on what you are able and willing to do, to get the best results possible.

Point Activation
There are several ways to activate the points. You can simply use your fingers and press on the points, which is the easiest

way, and it works. If you would like to try other methods, a good option is a mini massager. These massagers are about $10.

They have multiple heads to choose from. I have experimented with them and found the head with the most prongs on it is the strongest for acupressure.

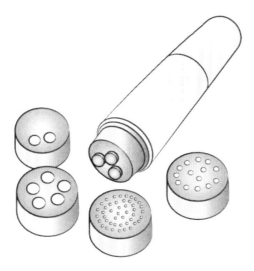

Vaccaria Seeds

Vaccaria seeds are another option to stimulate the points. This is a seed placed on a small piece of tape. It is often used for ear acupressure, but it can be used on other points. Women often use acupressure wristbands on Pericardium 6 to relieve nausea during pregnancy. I have seen other acupressure bands designed to treat other acupuncture points.

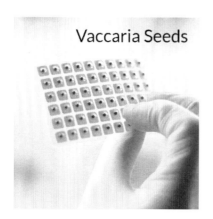

Vaccaria Seeds

The Body is Two Sided

The meridians are on both sides of the body, except the ones that go down the middle of your body. You can treat both sides, or just choose one. If you are treating pain, sometimes it works better to treat the opposite side of the pain. That is because when you are injured, there is often a lot of swelling in the area. Treating an area that is swollen can aggravate it. Treating the opposite side will get the best results in that case.

How to Locate Acupressure Points

Acupuncture points are located by either using bones, anatomical areas such as the eyes of the knee, the elbow crease, the belly button, the inner ankle bone, and also by measuring up from these areas.

The location of points is determined by measuring a distance from a landmark. The measurements used are done using the patient's anatomy. So if you are treating a baby, you use their two cun, not yours. If you are a woman, treating a man who has bigger bones than you do, you can use his fingers to determine how much his two cun is compared to yours.

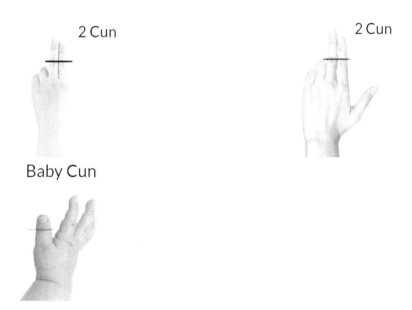

The first unit of measurement is called a cun. It is pronounced "soon." It is the width of your thumb joint.

1 Cun

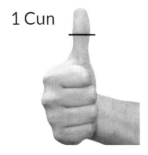

The next measurement is 2 cun, then 3 and 4 cun. If you need to count over 4 cun, you can add units as needed.

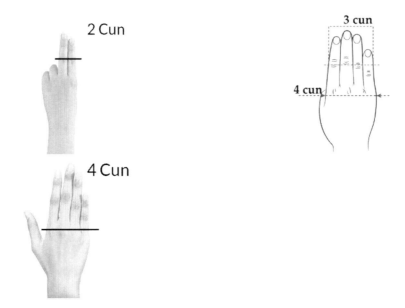

Be sure to use the same knuckle when you measure the points, and hold your hand in the correct position. For most points this will not matter, if it does matter, I mention it in the notes for each ailment. Pericardium 6 is often not measured correctly. The easiest way to locate it is using the 2 fingers measured up from the wrist crease.

You will notice that the location of the point can change when the position of the limb changes. You can try this on yourself by finding a point by holding your arm in a position that matches the image in this book. Circle the point, then move your arm in another direction, you will see how that can make it tricky to find. That is why each point is located with the limb in a precise position.

Photographs vs. Line Drawings

Most of the images in this book are photographs. Acupuncturists learn to locate points using line drawings that show the underlying bones, because we often use bony landmarks to locate points. I took an informal poll of my patients to find out if they preferred line drawings, or photographs with dots on them. They preferred the photographs. If the point location is tricky, I have included smaller line drawings next to the photos to make it clearer.

Cun Measurements

To make it an easy to use book, I have included the cun measurement images where needed. This will prevent you from having to flip back and forth in the book to remember what 2 cun is.

Point Diameter

Do not be too concerned about locating the point exactly. The points are not a pinhead size. You have leeway on your point location. Even if you are off a little, it is OK. The image below shows the idea of how large the point area is. That is also one reason why "sham acupuncture" often works. It is hard to avoid treating an acupuncture point, even if you try.

ST 36 Location

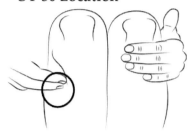

Diameter of Point

How Acupuncture and Acupressure Treat Pain

Acupuncture relieves pain in many ways. The first way is via the meridian system. The location of the pain is determined. The meridian that is affected is treated, which restores circulation in that meridian.

If you have arm pain, for example, we can often treat the Large Intestine meridian to resolve the pain. This meridian strongly restores circulation in the arm. Notice the pathway of the meridian from the end of the index finger to the nose. Any pain along that path can be treated by activating points on that meridian.

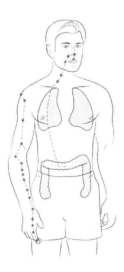

Large Intestine Meridian

In addition to treating pain via the affected meridian, other meridians can be treated that balance the meridian where the pain is located. So if the pain is on the Du meridian, the Ren meridian can be used to treat it.

There are other points that are used to treat pain. There are over 100 points on the body that treat back pain. That is because there are so many meridians that run through the back, that treating those meridians, or others that affect them, can restore circulation in the back.

It is not necessary for this to make sense to you to use acupressure points.

The Bladder meridian is often involved in back pain. You can see why when you see that there are two bladder lines on either side of the spine.

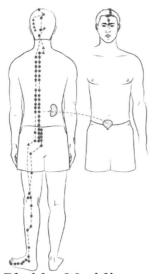

Bladder Meridian

You can see from the Gallbladder meridian image how both sciatica and migraines can both be caused by a blockage of that meridian. Notice how the meridian wraps around the side of the head, and also radiates from the hip all the way down the leg. That is a common location for sciatica.

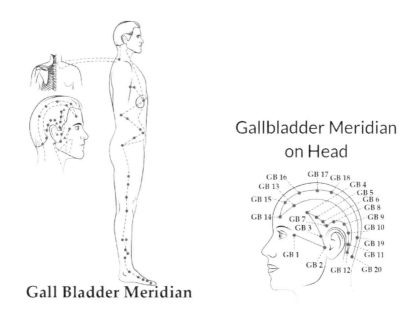

Gall Bladder Meridian

Gallbladder Meridian on Head

The Gallbladder meridian points on the foot can also be used to treat pain on the Gallbladder meridian points on the head.

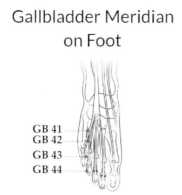

Gallbladder Meridian on Foot

Local Areas

In addition to using the meridian pathways to treat pain, treatment can be given on the area of pain. In Chinese medicine theory, pain is caused by blocked circulation. When circulation is restored, the tissue can receive enough oxygen and other nutrients to function normally. A tight muscle anywhere on the body can put pressure on nerves and blood vessels, which can hurt in another part of the body. That is why neck pain can be so damaging. The head has to get enough blood flow to be pain free.

If the neck muscles are tight, this can block healthy blood flow to the nerves that serve the ears, or anything on your head. If the neck and shoulders are tight, or causing pain, they should be treated to resolve any problem on the head.

You don't need to remember any of this information to use acupressure. I have chosen the most effective acupressure points for each type of pain. Some of the points that might be used for acupuncture might not be easily used for acupressure, so that is how I chose the easy to find, and most effective acupressure points.

Ear Acupressure Explained

Ear acupressure can be used to treat any type of ailment. It is especially popular to treat pain. All you have to do is look at an ear chart to determine where the body part is represented on the ear. You can apply a Vaccaria ear seed to that spot and press on it. The pellet will stay on the ear for a day or two and come off after you wash your hair. You should clean the point with alcohol before applying the seed.

When you press on the seed, be careful not to press too hard. Although it is not common, I have had a patient press so hard on her ear that it broke the skin. When the skin is broken, the area could get infected. Gentle pressure is all that is needed.

The human body is mapped on the ear and it looks like an upside down baby. There are different systems of ear acupuncture. The French have a system, and there is a Chinese system. As with acupuncture in general, there are many ways to treat a person. You can buy books about auricular acupuncture if you would like to delve into it further.

There are also pre-made ear acupressure kits that include the seeds and the ear maps to use them. It is easier to treat someone else, but not that hard to find the points to treat your own neck and back.

Ear Points Chart

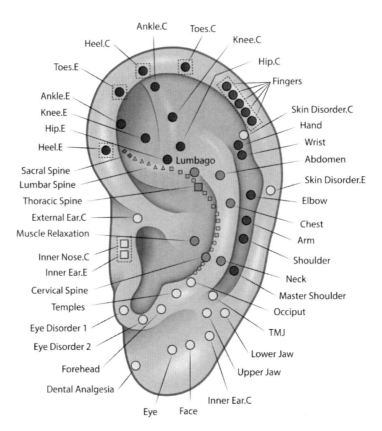

Ankle.C
Toes.C
Heel.C
Knee.C
Hip.C
Toes.E
Fingers
Ankle.E
Skin Disorder.C
Knee.E
Hand
Hip.E
Wrist
Heel.E
Abdomen
Lumbago
Sacral Spine
Lumbar Spine
Skin Disorder.E
Thoracic Spine
Elbow
External Ear.C
Chest
Muscle Relaxation
Arm
Inner Nose.C
Shoulder
Inner Ear.E
Neck
Cervical Spine
Master Shoulder
Temples
Occiput
Eye Disorder 1
TMJ
Eye Disorder 2
Lower Jaw
Forehead
Upper Jaw
Dental Analgesia
Inner Ear.C
Eye   Face

Vaccaria Seeds

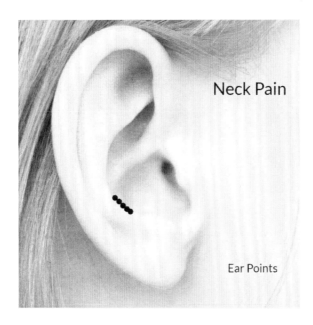

These are the points used to treat the neck. Please refer to the neck pain chapter for more information.

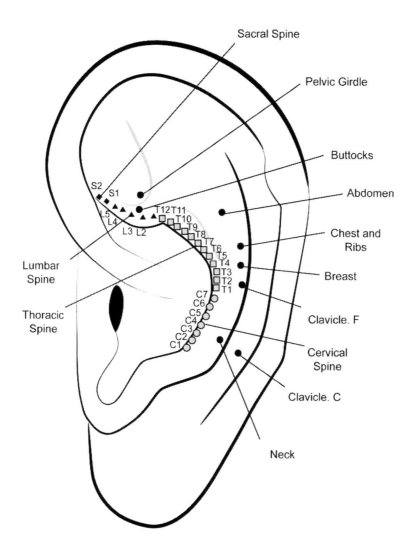

The cervical spine area corresponds to the neck. The thoracic spine corresponds to the mid-back, and the lumbar spine corresponds to the lower back.

When I treat the ear with acupressure pellets, I alternate ears. One treatment is the left ear, then the next is the right ear. The points will stop responding to the pellets, and they need a rest. You can get excellent results with this type of treatment.

If you read my acupuncture point book, *Acupuncture Points Handbook*, you will remember I had images of magnetic pellets and Sakamura pellets. I now just recommend Vaccaria seeds because they are easier to use. The seeds are larger and take less experience to apply them.

Acupuncture Meridians

There are 14 regular acupuncture meridians. You don't need to know where the meridians are located to do acupressure, but it is good to have a reference so you can see the correlation to the points, and the area affected.

The meridians are:
Bladder
Du or Governing Vessel
Gallbladder
Heart
Kidney
Large Intestine
Liver
Lung
Pericardium
Ren or Conception Vessel
Small Intestine
Spleen
Stomach
Triple Burner, Triple Warmer, or San Jiao

The Du meridian is also called the Governing Vessel, which is the English name. The Ren meridian is called the Conception Vessel in English. The Triple Burner channel is called the Triple Warmer, and the San Jiao meridian in Chinese.

Some meridians are commonly referred to by the Chinese name, others by the English name. You will see them both ways, depending on your reference and the author's preference. A meridian is also called a channel, it is the same thing, just different terminology.

Please note that I chose to clothe the images. So I covered up genitals and sensitive areas on the images. I did my best to make this a PG rated book. The woman in this section is wearing a bathing suit, and the man is wearing swim trunks.

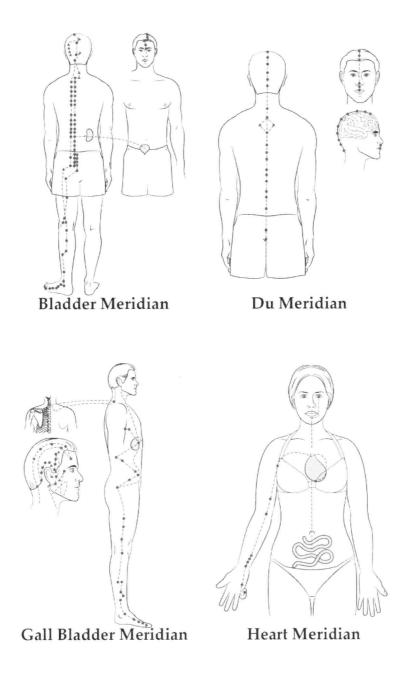

Bladder Meridian   Du Meridian

Gall Bladder Meridian   Heart Meridian

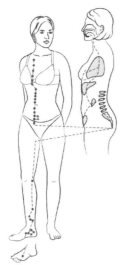

Kidney Meridian

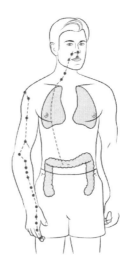

Large Intestine Meridian

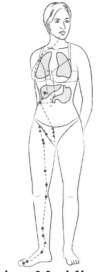

Liver Meridian

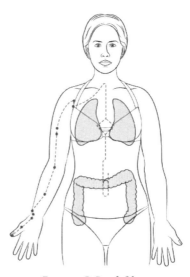

Lung Meridian

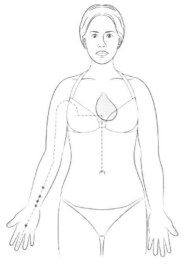

Pericardium Meridian

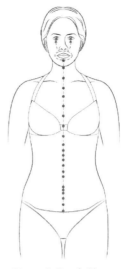

Ren Meridian

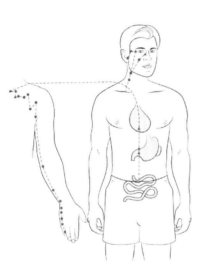

Small Intestine Meridian

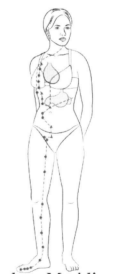

Spleen Meridian

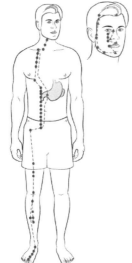

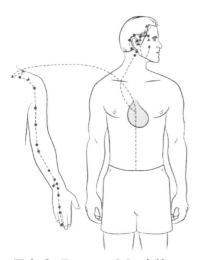

Stomach Meridian

Triple Burner Meridian

Acid Reflux or GERD, Gastroesophageal Reflux

Symptoms of acid reflux include burning pain in the chest or throat, regurgitating sour fluid, belching, difficulty swallowing, hiccups, and nausea. The reflux is often worse at night, and it can even cause insomnia. The acid can flow into the esophagus and damage the tissue, causing a partial obstruction.

Acid reflux is caused by a lack of stomach acid, not too much stomach acid. Taking drugs that suppress acid production in your stomach will not solve the problem.

If your digestion is healthy, and there is enough stomach acid, the sphincter at the top of your stomach will close and protect you from stomach acid seeping into your esophagus. If you do not have enough acid, the sphincter might not close, causing the acid to escape the stomach and leak into the esophagus.

Our goal with acupressure is to regulate and strengthen the stomach and intestines. If you are already taking acid blockers, please consult your doctor. Suddenly stopping these drugs can cause very serious rebound issues. Please allow enough time to resolve this problem, especially if you have already taken medications. This is a complicated matter and it is best to see an acupuncturist, because there are numerous causes and solutions to this problem.

Ren 12, 13, and 14 regulate the stomach, and diaphragm. Start with locating Ren 12 four cun above the belly button. Ren 13 is one cun above Ren 12, and Ren 14 is one cun above Ren 13.

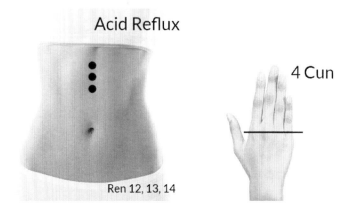

Acid Reflux

4 Cun

Ren 12, 13, 14

Pericardium 6 strongly regulates your stomach and heart area. It restores healthy circulation, treats nausea, and relieves pain. It is located with the wrist held flat, two cun from the wrist crease.

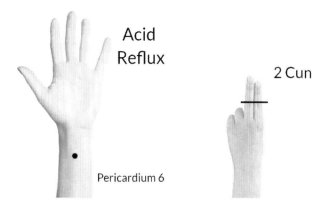

Acid Reflux

2 Cun

Pericardium 6

Stomach 36 is the number one point to boost energy levels, strengthen the immune system, and regulate and improve digestion. This point can treat any problem with the stomach.

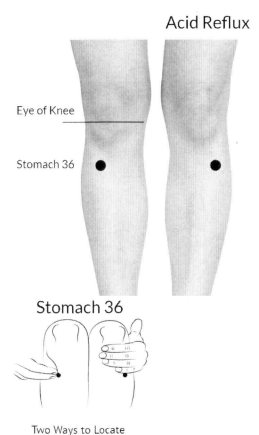

Acid Reflux

Eye of Knee

Stomach 36

Stomach 36

Two Ways to Locate

If you have treated yourself with acupressure and are not getting any relief, it is possible there is something else going on. A hiatal hernia is when part of the stomach is pushed up through the diaphragm. This is a physical problem, not an energetic one, so using acupressure points might not offer a lasting resolution. There are numerous videos online showing techniques for treating hiatal hernias.

Pressing in this area helps to relax tight tissue that causes congestion in the area. Simply press firmly. I have found breathing in and out quickly can help. Massage very firmly just below the ribs for a minute or two per point. I have found this technique to be effective. It is possible to find relief within minutes. Gently press beneath your ribcage, being careful around the xiphoid process, which is a little bone in the midline of your ribs.

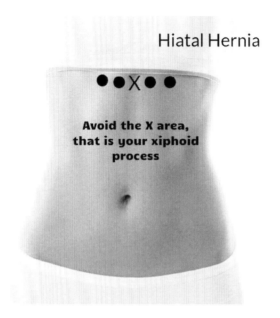

Acid reflux can cause insomnia. When you lie down the acid can leak into your esophagus and cause palpitations, which is when you feel your heart beating. If you are sleepy and go to bed, and after lying down you are wide awake or your heart is racing, it might be a hiatal hernia or acid reflux.

Treatment Notes
Since acid reflux is caused by a lack of stomach acid, you want to take herbs that increase stomach acid and improve digestion. Ginger root is very effective to increase stomach acid production. That alone might be all you need. It will take a little time to restore normal stomach function, but the good news is that ginger root is so effective for many ailments. It can be used to treat pain because it relieves inflammation. It also has been found to be more effective than anti-nausea drugs, with no side effects.

Ginger is the most important herb to keep at home. You can buy ground up ginger by Nature's Way or Solaray, or you can take a ginger root extract, which is made by boiling ginger root in water and dehydrating the liquid into a powder that is made into capsules and tablets. Jarrow makes a great ginger root extract product. Each capsule of the extract is equivalent to about 4 capsules of raw ginger. Planetary Herbals also has a good ginger root extract product in tablets. Some people drink ginger tea.

For fast relief of burning pain in the stomach, I like Acid Soothe by Enzymedica. If you ever have stomach problems, you should keep a bottle in your fridge. The burning is usually gone within minutes of taking it. I have not found any product to be as effective as this to stop burning pain. It has a special combination of ingredients that includes enzymes to improve digestion. Marshmallow root soothes the esophagus, stomach, and intestines. Papaya leaf, prickly ash, and others are also soothing. DGL licorice tablets are also helpful. Make sure the brand has 400 to 500 mg. of licorice root extract in it. One of my favorites changed the dosage recently. The one I now recommend is Natural Factors. It contains 400 mg. licorice root extract, and anise seed powder to improve digestion.

Allergies

Symptoms of allergies are nasal congestion, sneezing, clear nasal discharge, and itchy eyes. Common causes of allergic reactions are house dust, dust mite fecal matter, mold and mildew, animal dander, cigarette or cigar smoke, and perfumes.

The most important points for any allergic reaction are Large Intestine 4 and 11. These points strengthen the immune system and can reduce allergic reactions. For sinus symptoms, please see the sinus chapter for additional points. Pain on the face is often caused by sinus blockage.

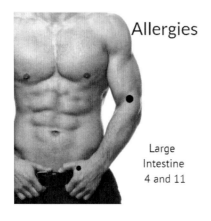

Allergies

Large Intestine 4 and 11

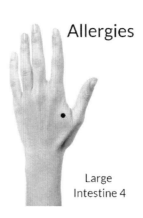

Allergies

Large Intestine 4

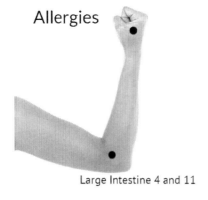

Allergies

Large Intestine 4 and 11

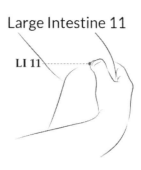

Large Intestine 11

LI 11

I got great results with these points doing acupressure, when I took a trip to Paris. A lot of people smoke in Paris. As I walked down the sidewalk I was exposed to a lot of smoke and I got sick every day. I did acupressure on these points daily and it calmed my immune system down within about an hour. They can help any type of allergic reaction.

Treatment Notes

There are popular herbal formulas that include herbs like astragalus and magnolia. Jade Windscreen is a popular formula that boosts the immune system to reduce allergies. I treated a little boy who was not able to go outside and play, due to his allergic reaction. I put him on an herbal formula called Jade Windscreen, and within about six weeks he had no problem going outside. Children respond very quickly. Some people have a reduction in allergies when they take probiotics.

Angina

Angina is chest pain. There are many causes of chest pain, and digestive problems often mimic the symptoms of angina. Your doctor should always be consulted for any type of chest pain.

I hesitated to include this information, because I was afraid people would treat themselves without consulting their doctor. However, I wanted to include information on how Chinese medicine treats angina. These acupuncture points are used to treat numerous causes of chest pain. For example, if you have chest pain caused by stomach problems Pericardium 6 will open the chest, which can treat problems caused by imbalances in the heart and stomach.

Heart 7 can be used to treat insomnia and anxiety, it also regulates the energy of the heart. Heart 5 is used to regulate the heart rhythm. Since Heart 5 is located one cun from Heart 7 you can treat both points at the same time.

Angina

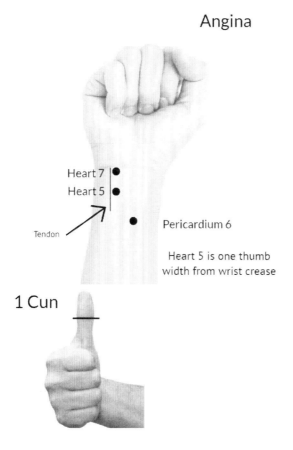

Heart 7

Heart 5

Tendon

Pericardium 6

Heart 5 is one thumb width from wrist crease

1 Cun

Treatment Notes

Hawthorn berry has been used as a gentle heart tonic for many years and is a prescribed medicine in Germany. Linus Pauling did research on how to treat clogged arteries with vitamin C, lysine, and proline.

Some people are resistant to this theory, so I will just mention it and you can decide for yourself. His theory was that plaque buildup in the arteries is caused by a vitamin C deficiency.

The body needs vitamin C to form healthy connective tissue. If there is not enough, the body has to work around it to repair the arteries. You might consider doing some research on this and speaking with your doctor about it.

A cardiologist, Dr. Stephen Sinatra, wrote a book called *Reverse Heart Disease Now*. He has been able to reverse heart disease with dietary changes, and nutritional supplements. He agrees with Dr. Pauling on his vitamin C theory and recommends additional supplements for the heart. When you do not have enough B vitamins, your homocysteine levels are too high. He says that homocysteine is a "prime causative agent in 20 to 40 percent of patients with arterial disease."

The heart supplements I often recommend to patients include:

- Jarrow Ubiquinol 400 mg per day.
- Garden of Life Raw multi-vitamins, they make the best absorbed vitamins you can buy. I can feel a difference between this brand and even my other favorite brands of vitamins. They are enzyme processed, so they are easily absorbed.
- Garden of Life Raw B vitamins. This is especially good for people with adrenal fatigue, which is caused by stress. Our body burns through B vitamins and vitamin C when we are under stress.
- Garden of Life Living vitamin C. This is a natural vitamin C, with all of the appropriate cofactors. Some people prefer all-natural vitamin C.
- Tru-OPC's from Nature's Way. This is a product researched and developed by Jacques Masquelier. He discovered an extract of grape seed that strengthens the veins and arteries and all connective tissue. It also improves the quality of your skin. I believe that strengthening blood vessels can help prevent numerous health problems, which can be caused by

weak blood vessels. Strokes and brain aneurisms for example, as well as varicose veins. My patients have bought cheaper brands of grape seed extract from discount and membership stores, but got no benefit at all. Just get the stuff that works!

- L-Carnitine helps your body burn fat for energy, balances blood sugar levels, and improves heart function. I like Jarrow Carnitine. Acetyl L-Carnitine is used to boost brain function.

- Krill oil helps keep your blood thinner and reduces inflammation. It is also good for your brain, as your brain is mostly fat. If you do not get enough Omega 3 oil, your brain will not function as well. Dr. Perricone has written many books about anti-aging, and he recommends fish oil as one of the most important supplements to take. Krill oil is easier to absorb, and unlikely to cause fish burp after you take it. Dr. Mercola was the first to promote krill oil over fish oil. Some people can take fish oil with no problem, but krill oil is more easily absorbed.

A friend of mine had a dog with a heart problem. Her vet told her that the dog would not survive very much longer. She gave the dog L-carnitine, CoQ10, and Cayenne pepper. The dog recovered and lived for many years. She put the supplements inside of a bit of meat, so he did not mind them.

Dick Quinn had bypass surgery and did not get any benefit from it. He wrote a book called *Left for Dead*. He used garlic and cayenne to clean out his arteries. He says that garlic softens the plaque, and cayenne makes the blood platelets slippery. I am not sure about the science behind it, but it is something to consider. I like Solaray Heart Blend SP-8. It has hawthorn berry, motherwort, rosemary, cayenne, kelp, wood betony, and shepherd's purse. Some people have a hard time taking cayenne at a full dose, but this product has other herbs in it to buffer the smaller amount of cayenne.

By no means am I suggesting you stop seeing your cardiologist or medical doctor. I just wanted to include this information so you will know that there are many natural solutions to health problems. Your doctor could not even suggest them, so you will need to do your own research. Just do not accept a death sentence from anyone. No one can tell you what is possible for you if you do not give up.

Ankle Pain

When acupuncturists treat pain, we first need to determine which area or meridian is affected. If the pain is on the front of your ankle, Stomach 41 is a good starting place. There is a little hollow in the top of the ankle, which is where the point is located.

Stomach 41 also treats foot drop, foot pain, and lower leg pain, atrophy, and stiffness.

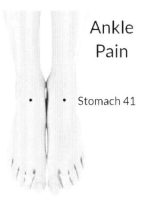

Ankle
Pain

• Stomach 41

Spleen 5 is located on the inside of the ankle, below the inner ankle bone. This point treats ankle and foot pain. It is a good choice to treat pain on the inner ankle. Since Spleen 6 is a major point for excess fluid, and the main point on the meridian, you could treat that also.

Ankle Pain

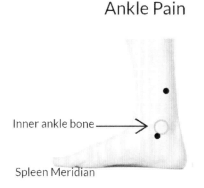

Inner ankle bone

Spleen Meridian

Gallbladder 40 is located in front of and below the outer ankle bone. It treats ankle pain, foot drop, rib pain, wrist pain, and lower back pain. It treats pain on the outer ankle.

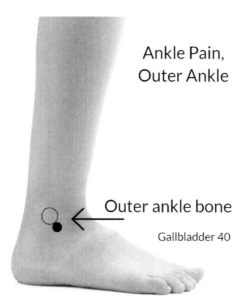

Ankle Pain,
Outer Ankle

Outer ankle bone

Gallbladder 40

Treatment Notes

A mini massager would work best. If the ankles are swollen, you can treat the kidneys and spleen, which helps your body get rid of excess fluid. Please refer to the chapter on water retention for more information.

Anxiety

Chinese medicine is amazing to treat emotional issues. Emotional health and physical health go hand in hand. Emotional issues have a root in physical issues. The physical imbalance can be treated with acupuncture and Chinese herbs, which will resolve the emotional issues.

The number one point to treat anxiety is Heart 7. This calms the mind. Pericardium 6 is also a good option. Both of these points treat insomnia and anxiety. Pericardium 6 is 2 cun from the wrist crease, in the middle of the arm.

Anxiety

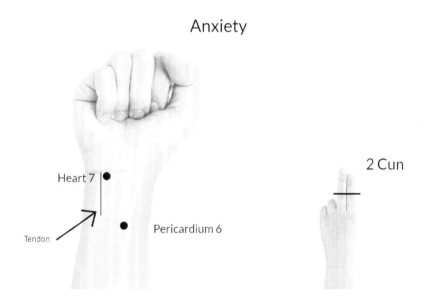

If stress is causing your anxiety, it is helpful to treat the liver. In Chinese medicine theory, stress affects the liver, and treating the liver relieves stress. Liver 3 treats stress and anxiety. Liver 3 is the number one point to treat stress. Sometimes it is hard to tell the difference between stress and anxiety, since stress often causes anxiety, so treating the liver is a good option. Run your fingers in the area and you will find a small dip between the toes. That is where Liver 3 is located.

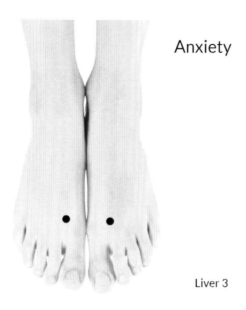

Anxiety

Liver 3

Spleen 6 is very calming. It regulates the hormones, treats insomnia, and is helpful for anxiety and stress.

Anxiety

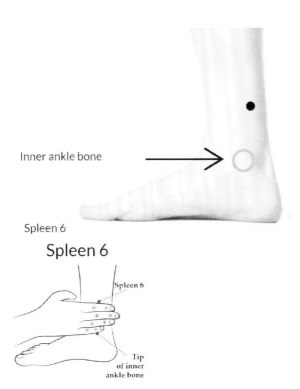

Inner ankle bone

Spleen 6

Spleen 6

Spleen 6

Tip
of inner
ankle bone

Treatment Notes

There are many Chinese herbal formulas that treat anxiety. They address a heart deficiency, which is often at the root of the problem.

Gotu kola, which is also called *centella asiatica*, is my favorite over the counter herb for stress and anxiety. It is an Indian herb. It improves memory and focus. It also strengthens the veins, and has been used to treat skin disorders. Nature's Way and Solaray are the brands I use, I usually suggest 3 capsules at a time, once a day.

Bach Flower Remedies Rescue Remedy is very helpful to treat stress and anxiety. It is the extract of flowers, which treats emotional issues.

Arm Pain

Acupuncture points can be used to relieve pain, but they also can be used to improve the healing of broken bones. Treat the points on the opposite side of the broken bone.

The body is bilateral, which means you can treat either side. If you have a broken bone, treat the opposite side points several times a day to improve blood flow and speed healing.

When treating pain, the first choice is to treat the strongest points. On the arm, Large Intestine 4, 11, and 15 are the strongest for the arm. Stimulating these points will restore healthy circulation in the arm. They are often included to treat any problem on the arm, such as elbow and hand pain.

These points can also be used for recovery after a stroke. Please see the stroke section for more information.

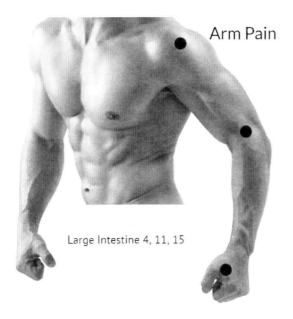

Arm Pain

Large Intestine 4, 11, 15

Sometimes arm pain can originate in the spine. When the muscles are tight in the neck and upper back, this disrupts blood flow to the arm. Feel for tender spots on the shoulders, and treat them with massage.

Baby Acupressure

Babies only need very light stimulation of the points. I do not recommend the mini massager or any other type of stimulation. Always consult your doctor before treatment.

It is sometimes hard to determine what the diagnosis is with adults, and especially so with children. The beauty of acupressure and Chinese medicine in general is that all you need to do is stimulate the points of the affected body part, and the body regulates itself.

It is not necessary to have a precise Western diagnosis. It is nice to have, but if you have a stomach problem, you treat the stomach. If you have a constipation problem, you treat the large intestine meridian, which regulates the colon. I would always consult a medical doctor to rule out something serious, before I attempted acupressure on a baby.

Baby Bedwetting

This bedwetting section applies to a child of any age. I have placed it in the baby section so it is easy to find to treat children.

Bedwetting in children is most commonly caused by the same thing as incontinence or frequent urination in adults, a kidney energy weakness. The kidneys are responsible for the ability to retain the urine and stool.

A child inherits her kidney strength from her mother. Women lose kidney energy when they carry and give birth to babies. That is why there is a tradition in Chinese medicine to treat the mother after she gives birth. Women take Chinese herbal medicine to restore lost blood and restore energy levels.

If a woman gives birth to many children it depletes her kidneys. I believe this is a common cause of postpartum depression. All of this is treatable with Chinese medicine.

The kidneys can be strengthened using points on the kidney meridian. The most important points to use are Kidney 3 and 7.

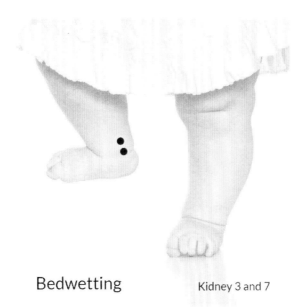

Bedwetting   Kidney 3 and 7

Treatment Notes

Herbs are very helpful to strengthen the kidneys and restore bladder strength. Cordyceps is an effective kidney tonic. There are dozens of herbal formulas that can be used to boost the kidneys.

In acupuncture school I treated a little boy who wet the bed. He took kidney tonic herbs and his mom did acupressure on him and within a few months he no longer wet the bed. Since he inherited a kidney weakness from his mother who had weak kidneys from having so many children, it took longer for him to recover than it usually does for children.

Baby Colds and Flu

Colds and flu can turn into pneumonia and bronchitis if not treated. Please consult your medical doctor to be sure you are doing everything you can and the baby is evaluated regularly.

When the body is invaded by a cold or flu virus, the body produces excess mucus to protect itself. In Chinese medicine, we do not dry mucus when a patient has an active cold or flu. Drying the mucus membranes can drive the virus deeper and prevent the body from protecting itself.

However, mucus can build up and get infected and turn into an upper respiratory infection, pneumonia, and many other lung conditions. It is better to take antiviral and antibacterial herbs, rather than to dry mucus.

Acupressure can be used to boost the immune system, reduce a fever, reduce coughing, and reduce mucus naturally. There is actually an acupuncture point that is called the "Phlegm Point." It helps the body to resolve mucus.

Treatments can be given every hour or two. In most cases, the more often you treat these points, the faster the person will recover. When the points are stimulated, it boosts the immune system to dispel the virus.

Large Intestine 4 is one of the top acupuncture points. It is called the face point, because it can be used to treat the face. It also boosts the immune system and reduces allergies. It treats ear infections, headaches, and hives. It regulates the lungs, treats sinus congestion, sore throat, toothache, nosebleed, and regulates sweating.

Colds and Flu

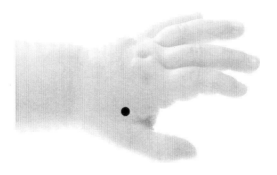

Large Intestine 4

Large intestine 11 is used to boost the immune system and reduce a fever. It is the number one point to reduce fevers. It is located on the crease by the elbow. It is also used to treat constipation and clear inflammation in the large intestine. I once used this point to reduce the fever in a patient in her seventies. She had become delirious and this point brought down her fever within an hour.

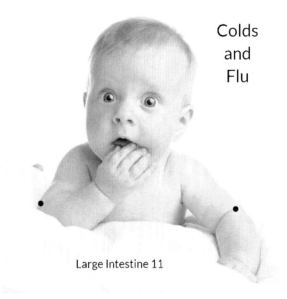

Colds
and
Flu

Large Intestine 11

Stop Coughing

Lung 7 is the best choice to stop coughing. It works by regulating and strengthening the lungs. It also helps resolve mucus or phlegm in the lungs or sinuses, and treats wheezing. Lung 7 can be tricky to find on a baby. The point is located on the bone, about 2 fingers from the wrist.

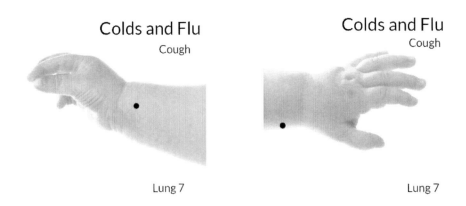

Colds and Flu
Cough

Lung 7

Colds and Flu
Cough

Lung 7

Lung 5 is in the inner elbow crease. It is easier to find the point with the elbow flexed, making a fist, but that will be hard to do on a baby. Just make sure you locate the point on the thumb side of the arm. You should be able to locate the bicep tendon. Lung 5 clears heat or inflammation from the lungs, treats cough, inflammatory lung conditions, regulates the lung function, and treats shortness of breath and wheezing.

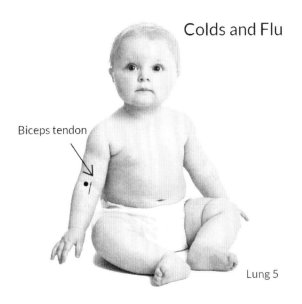

Colds and Flu

Biceps tendon

Lung 5

Stomach 36 has over 50 indications. It regulates and strengthens digestion, regulates the intestines, strengthens the immune system and many other things. For cold and flu it is used to regulate and strengthen the lungs. It is used for asthma, cough, fatigue, and breathing difficulty. It is located just below the knee.

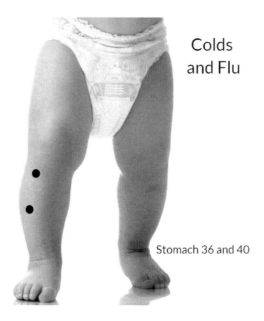

Colds
and Flu

Stomach 36 and 40

Stomach 40 is known as the phlegm point. It resolves mucus of any type. It helps the body resolve mucus in colds and flu, as well as allergies. It treats chest pain from lung issues, asthma, bronchitis, coughing, wheezing, and pneumonia.

When I use Stomach 40 on patients with a cold, they often start coughing after I remove the needles. I see this as a good response. That shows how the point is making their body get rid of mucus in the lungs. It is a productive cough. It is located halfway down the calf. In adults it is about two finger widths away from the tibia bone, or shin bone. In a baby, just find the bone and press very close to it.

Treatment Notes
There are many herbs that treat viruses. Echinacea liquid extract, elderberry extract by Sambucol can be helpful. There are herbal formulas designed to be given to children.

Baby Colic

Symptoms of colic can include: Pain or discomfort from gas or indigestion, underfeeding or overfeeding, and a sensitivity to formula or breast milk. It is not known what causes colic.

As an acupuncturist, I would address the probable causes. There might be several causes. I would start first with regulating the colon to ensure good bowel movements and reduced gas.

Large Intestine 11 regulates the colon and relieves constipation, and is used to relieve intestinal "heat" or inflammation in the intestines. Babies usually respond within minutes to acupressure on this point. They will have a bowel movement. If that relieves them and they calmed down, the problem is solved.

Colic

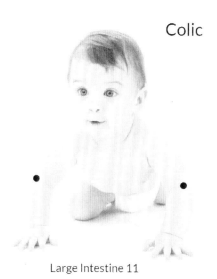

Large Intestine 11

If that did not relieve the problem, I would work my way up and treat the digestion. There are several points that regulate the stomach and intestines. These points are used to improve digestion, and regulate the stomach and intestines.

Stomach 36 is the next option. This point also boosts the immune system and improves digestion. This is one of the most important points on the body.

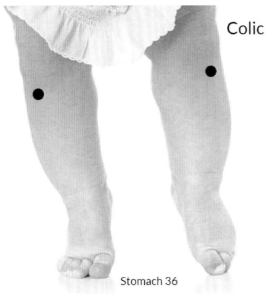

Colic

Stomach 36

I would treat Stomach 36 on both sides, for five to ten minutes.

The next option is regulating the stomach. These points are the same ones used to treat acid reflux in adults. Ren 12 and Ren 13.

Ren 12 is located about the width of your baby's fist above the belly button. Ren 13 is one finger above that. On a baby you will be treating both at the same time as the points are very small.

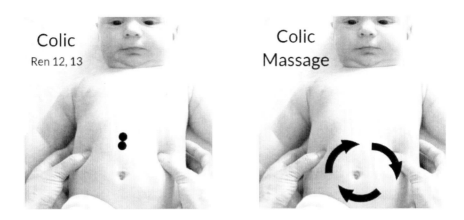

Colic
Ren 12, 13

Colic
Massage

A common practice in some countries is to massage the baby's belly in a clockwise motion. This encourages the colon to function properly. You can find many videos online doing this.

Treatment Notes
A good option would be children's probiotics. Children often do not have enough good bacteria in their intestines to be healthy. Consider the diet. Wheat can be very constipating and irritating to the intestines. I have heard stories of breastfeeding mothers stopping all dairy products and getting good results. Dairy protein is a common allergen in babies and adults. Humans do not have the enzymes necessary to digest cow's milk. That is why it can cause excess mucus production, allergies, coughing, and sneezing. It is an allergen.

Baby Cun

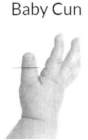

Baby Constipation

Treating constipation in babies is very easy. They usually respond to acupressure within minutes. There is only one point you need to know, Large Intestine 11. This point regulates and moistens the large intestine, which relieves constipation. It helps to restore normal bowel function. This point can be used as often as needed, at least once daily until the large intestine has been regulated.

If digestion is weak, I would add Stomach 36 to strengthen and regulate all aspects of digestion and elimination.

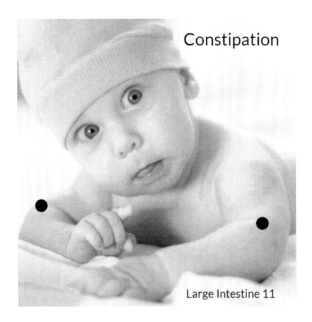

Constipation

Large Intestine 11

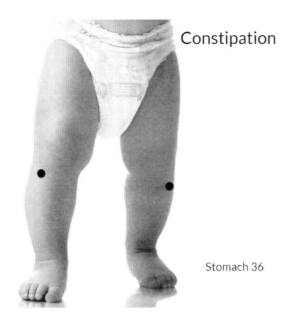

Constipation

Stomach 36

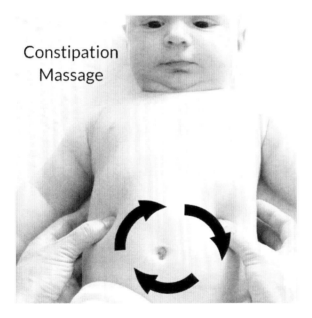

Constipation
Massage

Another option that has been used for centuries to restore normal colon function is abdominal massage. You gently massage the baby's abdomen around the navel in a clockwise motion. This is how the large intestine normally functions. This massage is often done about 50 times.

Constipation

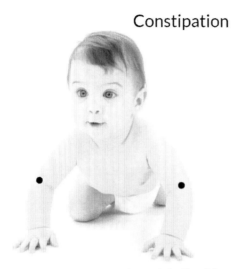

Large Intestine 11

Baby Diarrhea

Diarrhea is treated using points that regulate digestion, as well as points that improve digestion.

Stomach 36 is the most important point to use. It strengthens and regulates the stomach and intestines. Stomach 37 treats diarrhea, gastritis, and intestinal abscess. Stomach 36 is located just below the kneecap. Stomach 37 is located 3 cun below Stomach 36.

Stomach 25 is located 2 cun away from the navel. It treats diarrhea, constipation, vomiting, and colitis by regulating the intestinal function.

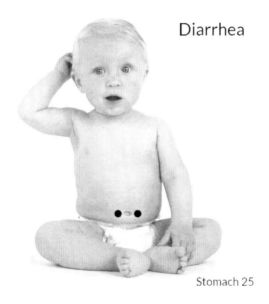

Diarrhea

Stomach 25

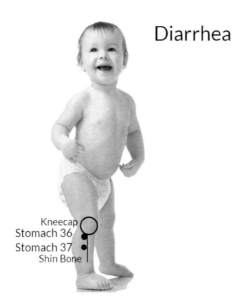

Diarrhea

Kneecap
Stomach 36
Stomach 37
Shin Bone

Treatment Notes

Ginger root is what I recommend for adults to treat diarrhea. Good probiotics can also help treat diarrhea. Many companies now make powdered probiotics for children.

Baby Digestion

The main point to strengthen digestion is stomach 36. This point can be treated daily to improve health.

The size of Stomach 36 is very large. It is very difficult to miss it. It is located on the outside of the leg, just below the knee.

This point can be used often to strengthen and regulate digestion. It also strengthens the immune system, and regulates the intestines to treat intestinal issues.

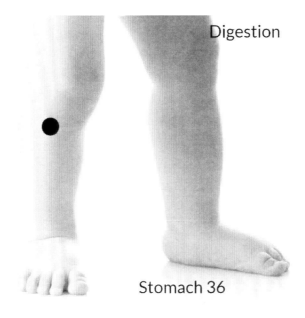

Digestion

Stomach 36

Baby Ear Pain

As with all ailments, you should consult with your pediatrician before trying acupressure.

Points around the ear restore healthy blood flow and relieve ear pain. Pain is caused by a lack of blood circulation in the affected area. Anything that improves circulation can relieve pain. Ear infections are caused by viruses and bacteria. The body needs to resolve the problem via a healthy immune system.

Triple Warmer 21 is at the root of the ear. It is used to open and regulate the ears. It restores normal ear circulation to treat ear disorders.

Gallbladder 2 opens the ears to treat deafness, tinnitus, ear infections and discharge, as well as ear pain, jaw pain, and TMJ pain.

Small Intestine 19 is located in front of the ear. It treats ear discharge and inflammation, and vertigo due to ear problems.

Triple Warmer 17 is located behind the earlobe. It relieves pain, treats itching inside the ear, pain and swelling of the ear, earache, and tinnitus.

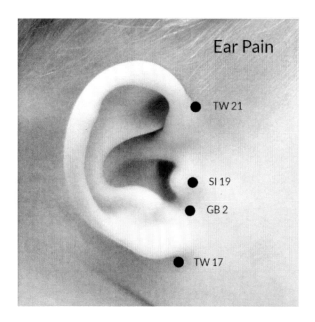

To fight off bacteria and viruses, the immune system needs to be strong. I would treat Large Intestine 4 and 11 to boost the immune system. Gentle pressure on both sides for about 5 minutes should be all that is needed.

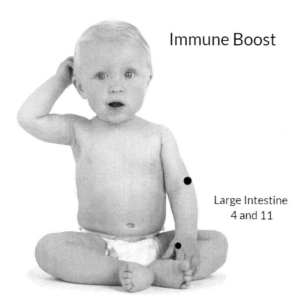

Immune Boost

Large Intestine
4 and 11

Stomach 36 is important to improve the immune system and digestion.

Treatment Notes
Treating the virus or bacteria topically with garlic ear oil can be helpful. Garlic kills bacteria. Astragalus is a deep immune tonic often given to children in China to improve digestion and immunity. Planetary Herbals makes an astragalus extract in liquid form. The Herbs for Kids brand also has an astragalus liquid.

Hyland's makes a homeopathic ear drop called Infant Earache drops. Herb Pharm Kids has a product with mullein, garlic oil, calendula, and St. John's Wort.

Astragalus root extract can be taken regularly to boost the immune system. Good probiotics would also improve the immune system, which is especially important if antibiotics have already been taken.

Baby Fever

Fever is produced by your body to kill viruses and bacteria. Consult your doctor for any type of fever. Large intestine 11 is used to reduce fever. This point is located by the elbow and it is used for allergies, and cold and flu. It is located on the elbow crease.

Any type of fever can be treated using this point. It can also be used to treat hives and other skin disorders caused by inflammation.

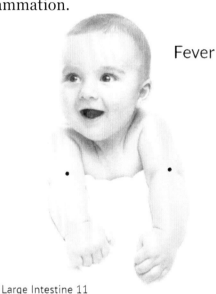

Fever

Large Intestine 11

Baby Sleep

If a baby cannot sleep, you have to determine why. If there are intestinal problems, or digestive problems, they should be treated. Please see the chapter on colic to treat intestinal issues. If the baby has colic, that should be treated first.

For general soothing, there are several good options. These points can be used for any emotional upset.

Heart 7 treats anxiety and insomnia. It calms the mind to help you get to sleep and stay asleep. This point is located at the wrist crease.

Sleep

Heart 7,
and Pericardium 6

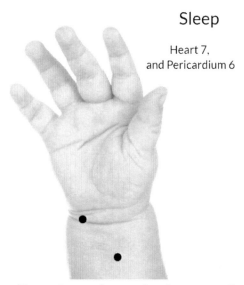

Pericardium 6 regulates the heart and stomach, which can help with digestive issues also. It calms the stomach, treats anxiety, hiccups, vomiting, and any type of nausea.

Yin Tang can be translated as "Spirit Gate." It calms the mind, and treats insomnia. It is located between the eyes.

Sleep

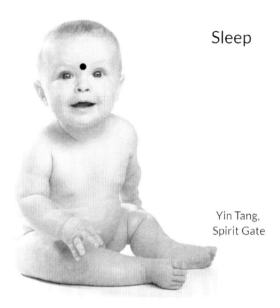

Yin Tang,
Spirit Gate

Spleen 6 is a very calming point. It pulls energy down to the feet, so it should not be used by pregnant women. It is one hand width above the inner ankle bone, using the baby's hand size.

Sleep

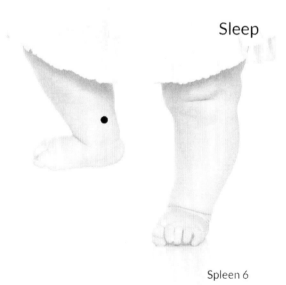

Spleen 6

Another good option is Kidney 6. This point also is very calming. It treats insomnia and it should not be used by pregnant women, because it expedites labor. Although I have discussed this with numerous acupuncturists and the consensus is that in most cases, no matter what you do, the baby comes when it wants to. Relaxing the mother is the primary objective. Kidney 6 is located just below the inner ankle bone on the inside of the foot.

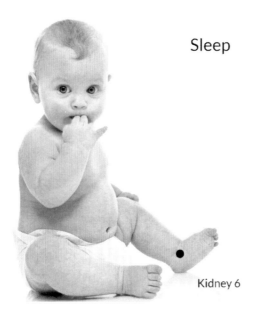

Sleep

Kidney 6

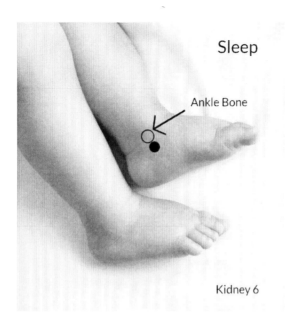

Sleep

Ankle Bone

Kidney 6

Kidney 1 is on the bottom of the foot. It calms the mind, treats anxiety, insomnia, and headache. It pulls energy down from the head. It is one of the strongest points on the body to calm someone down.

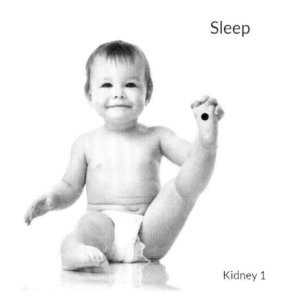

Sleep

Kidney 1

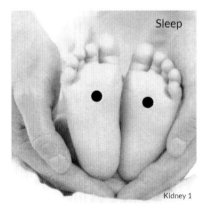

If you feel your baby is stressed out, Liver 2 and 3 are very relaxing. These two points are two of the most commonly used points in acupuncture. They are very calming, and most people need them. The most commonly used point is Liver 3. I would just gently massage between the toes in that area.

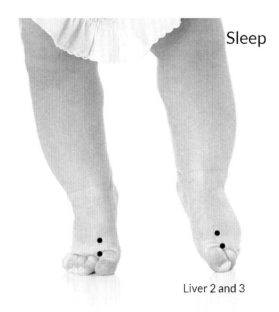

Treatment Notes

One of my favorite supplements for insomnia is Bach Flower Remedies. They are safe to use. They should not be confused with essential oils. Essential oils are the flower oils and are not usually consumed. Flower essences are made by putting the flowers in water and extracting them. This is not homeopathy, although the percentage of flower essences is a minute amount.

Bach Rescue Sleep and Bach Rescue Remedy are very calming. My patients often say they feel like they took a sedative after they take Bach Rescue Sleep. This is not a sedative, it helps to relax the mind. There is a child version of this formula also. The difference is that it is alcohol free, although the amount of alcohol in the adult version is miniscule and I have not known anyone to react to it.

Just spritz it a few times in the mouth. If the insomnia is caused by emotional issues, this will help a lot. Rescue Remedy is used to treat stress and anxiety.

Baby Stress

Stress affects all of us. Liver 3 is the best point to treat stress. I would consider also treating Spleen 6, because it is a very calming point.

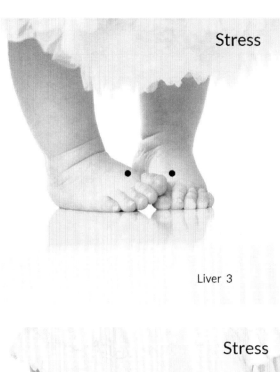

Stress

Liver 3

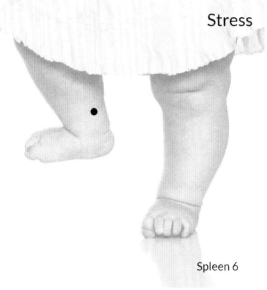

Stress

Spleen 6

Treatment Notes

Bach Rescue Remedy is available for children. It is a flower essence formula that is very calming.

Baby Vomiting

Vomiting can be caused by many things, so after seeing your medical doctor, you can try regulating the stomach and intestines with acupressure.

Vomiting can be caused by a viral infection, including the common cold and flu.

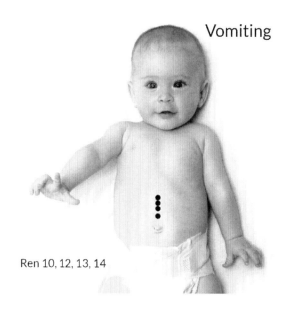

Vomiting

Ren 10, 12, 13, 14

Points Ren 10, 12, 13, and 14 are used to regulate the stomach and intestines. You can apply gentle finger pressure to the points, but perhaps a gentle massage downward would be more helpful. In Chinese medicine theory, the stomach energy is supposed to go down. When it is not going down, it can cause nausea. So stimulating the stomach to function normally is encouraging it to send the energy down.

Vomiting caused by a cold or flu should be treated by the points in that chapter. The most important points to treat for any immune issue are Large Intestine 4 and 11. Large intestine 11 treats fevers and constipation, it also regulates the intestines. Large intestine 4 strengthens the immune system.

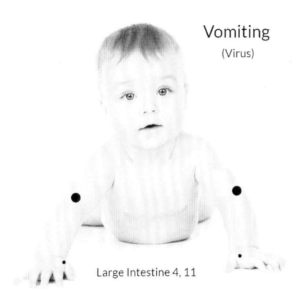

Large Intestine 4, 11

Pericardium 6 is two cun from the wrist crease and it regulates the stomach to relieve vomiting.

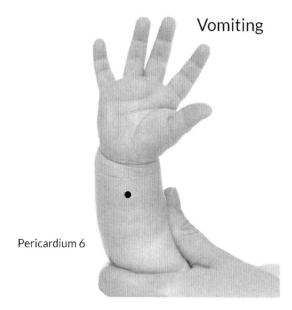

Vomiting

Pericardium 6

Stomach 36 strengthens and regulates the stomach and intestines. It is located just below the outer kneecap.

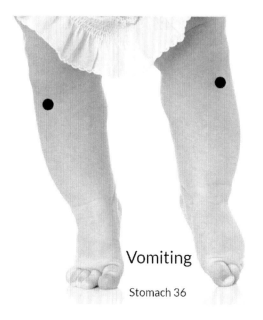

Vomiting

Stomach 36

Back Pain

There are over 100 acupuncture points that treat back pain. Some are located on the back, but many are located on the hands and feet. It is very easy to treat yourself, and surgery is rarely necessary. My book, *Natural Back Pain Solutions*, includes information on supplements, stretches, and an in-depth discussion on this.

My favorite acupressure point for back pain is called Ling Gu. This point is in the Tung acupuncture system, which is a different system of acupuncture.

Every acupuncturist is a pain specialist. We treat back pain from our first day in student clinic. Whether your back pain is caused by tight muscles, pinched nerves, or herniated discs, acupuncture is a solution.

The best way to treat this point is by using a mini massager. I have personally done acupressure on this point, and found it to be very effective. Press very firmly into the joint with the massager. Ling Gu is located on the hand, between the thumb and index finger bones. I have included an image that shows the hand bones.

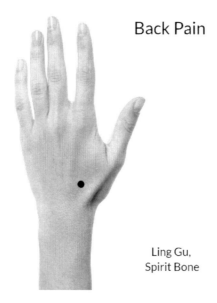

Back Pain

Ling Gu,
Spirit Bone

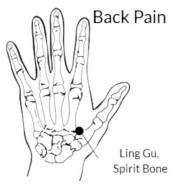

Back Pain

Ling Gu,
Spirit Bone

Lower back pain can be associated with a kidney energy weakness in Chinese medicine. Treating the kidneys treats the lower back.

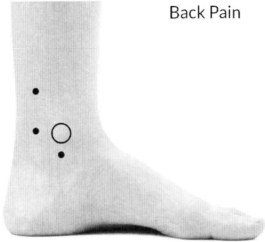

Back Pain

Kidney 3, 6, 7

Treat Where It Hurts

Most of the back pain patients I treat have very tight back muscles, and they have tiny knots in their backs. This is what happens when you have muscle pain a long time. The muscle seems to have knots in it. I insert needles into the knots and the knots relax. Acupuncture works very fast to resolve this.

Treatment Notes

Tight muscles are the most common cause of back pain. Acupuncture quickly relaxes tight muscles. Some people get back surgery thinking it is a herniated disc that is causing the pain, when it is simply tight muscles. This is easily treated by acupuncture.

With chronic back pain, over time the muscles get tighter and tighter and they can feel like knots. I think everyone who is considering getting back surgery should get acupuncture first. In some cases, patients recover within 10 visits. That is a complete cure of back pain.

If you have a herniated disc, supplements can help. Your body uses joint supplements like type two collagen, glucosamine sulfate, chondroitin sulfate, and MSM to repair a herniated disc or any joint issue. I like the Jarrow brand, and the Doctor's Best brand. The quality of the supplements you take is very important.

I know it can be difficult if you do not buy a lot of supplements to be familiar with some of the best brands. That is why I include the brand names. I have tried many brands over 20 years now and I know what gets results quickly. If you bought a joint supplement from a discount store and did not get results, you might consider buying one of the brands I recommend and see if that makes a difference.

Carpal Tunnel Syndrome

Carpal tunnel syndrome is an inflammation of the nerve in the wrist. Often the tendon that holds down the wrist tendons is inflamed, and swells, which blocks the normal nerve function to the hand.

It is not uncommon for people to get a diagnosis of carpal tunnel when in fact it is something else. In order to treat hand pain, you need to know if it is true carpal tunnel, or pain originating elsewhere, such as thoracic outlet syndrome, inflamed nerves, or a wrist joint inflammation.

Pericardium 6 is located near the carpal tunnel. Using a mini massager on this point will restore healthy blood flow so the body can treat the inflammation. Inflammation is the body treating to heal itself. Restoring healthy blood flow will enable your body to heal.

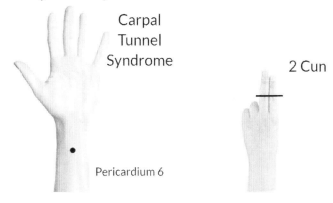

Carpal Tunnel Syndrome

2 Cun

Pericardium 6

If the shoulders are tight, Gallbladder 21 can help relax them. If this is not enough, please see the shoulder pain protocol and treat the shoulders also. The shoulders can get tight and this can put too much pressure on the nerves, which causes a disruption of normal nerve function.

If I had carpal tunnel syndrome, I would include acupressure massages along the sides of the spine, on the neck muscles, and points at the top of the shoulder.

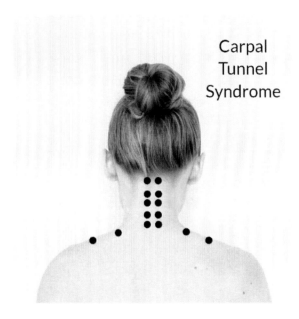

Carpal
Tunnel
Syndrome

A common cause of carpal tunnel is not sitting correctly, or standing all day and not paying attention to posture. This tightens the neck and shoulder muscles, which can put pressure on the nerves that go down the arms. It is very easy to slump over when you are supposed to sit in one position all day.

Carpal Tunnel Syndrome

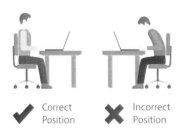

Correct Position   Incorrect Position

In my experience, carpal tunnel syndrome is the diagnosis you will get if you have any repetitive stress injury. You could have thoracic outlet syndrome also. Stretching and treating the neck and shoulders will go a long way to relieving this problem.

Treatment Notes

For relief of inflammation enzymes such as bromelain and FYI Restore can be used. They should be taken on an empty stomach. If the only problem is an inflammation of the tendon, enzymes should be effective, as they treat the root cause of inflammation. If the shoulders are tight or you sit at a desk all day and do not stretch your shoulders, you might needs to do shoulder stretches.

If there is a nerve entrapment causing the pain, treating the wrist will not be effective enough. I would also consider Thermacare heat patches to relax the neck and shoulder muscles. These patches can be worn all day.

If you sit at a desk all day, doing shoulder stretches and getting up and walking around is important. The images below are my favorite stretches for carpal tunnel and thoracic outlet syndrome.

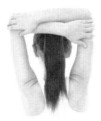

Carpal
Tunnel
Stretch

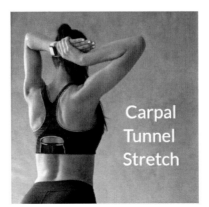

Carpal
Tunnel
Stretch

Carpal Tunnel

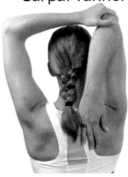

Carpal Tunnel Syndrome

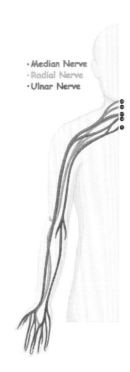

- Median Nerve
- Radial Nerve
- Ulnar Nerve

Cold and Flu

Points that boost the immune system are extremely effective to speed recovery from a cold or flu. The most important points to treat are Large Intestine 4 and 11, Stomach 36 and 40, and Lung 7.

Large Intestine 4 and 11 are the first points to choose for any immune problem. They treat allergies and sinus also. Large Intestine 11 reduces a fever.

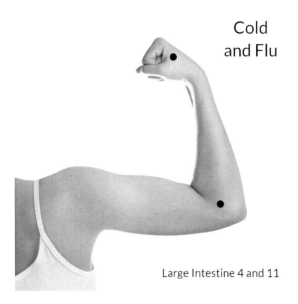

Cold and Flu

Large Intestine 4 and 11

Lung 5 is only necessary if the cold has caused lung symptoms like wheezing, bronchitis, and lung shortness of breath. These are serious symptoms and you should see an MD immediately. I am including this point so you can treat it after you see an MD.

Cold and Flu

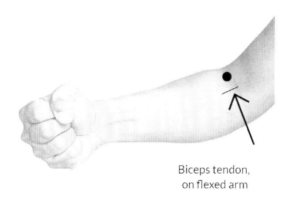

Biceps tendon,
on flexed arm

Lung 5

Lung 5 can be located by flexing the arm to find the bicep tendon. The point is on the thumb side of the tendon.

If you make a mistake and treat the other side of the tendon, it is no problem. Although I don't use this point for colds, it is Pericardium 3, which regulates the heart, and restores circulation in the chest to treat hives and fever.

Lung 7 is my first choice to stop coughing. It treats wheezing, bronchitis, and helps resolve mucus in the lungs. It also strengthens the lungs, which will help your body fight off the virus. It can easily be located by placing the hands together and finding the indentation at the end of the fingertip.

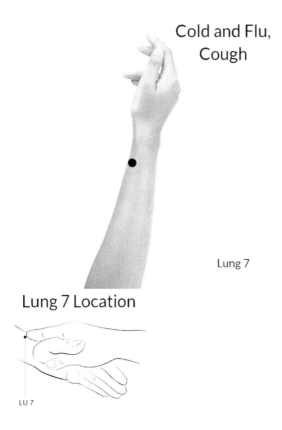

Cold and Flu,
Cough

Lung 7

Lung 7 Location

LU 7

When I was in acupuncture school my dad had a cold and it had turned into a barking cough. I knew that meant that he was not clearing the virus, and it was going internal and would possibly turn into bronchitis or pneumonia. He was not a believer in acupuncture back then, but he put up with my treating him every two hours or so. I simply treated Large Intestine 4, 11, Stomach 36, 40, and Lung 7. The next day he was not coughing at all.

Stomach 36 boosts your immune system and energy levels. Stomach 40 is known as the Phlegm Point. It helps to resolve excess mucus anywhere in the body. Stomach 40 is in the middle of the calf bone, as measured from the eye of the knee and the outer ankle bone. Another way to measure it is about 8 cun down from the eye of the knee. Find the top of the shin bone, and the point is 2 cun from that.

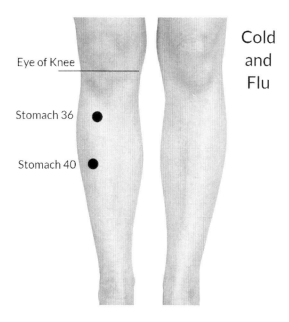

Stomach 40 Location

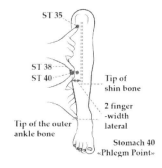

Treatment Notes
There are Chinese herbal formulas developed in modern times to treat viruses. If I were not able to use the formulas available only through acupuncturists, I would take Planetary Herbals Andrographis Respiratory Wellness. The ingredients are: Andrographis Aerial Parts Extract, Olive

Leaf Extract, *Echinacea purpurea* Root Extract, Isatis Root Extract, Goldenseal Root, Dandelion Root Extract, Garlic Bulb, Ginger Root, and Licorice Root. This formula will kill all types of viruses. I use a formula similar to this to treat bladder infections, and other types of infections. If herbal formulas like this are taken at the first sign of a cold or flu, it can often be resolved very quickly before you get very sick.

There is a book about the many herbs that treat different types of viruses. The book is *Herbal Antivirals*, by Stephen Harrod Buhner. I use this book regularly. Stephen even includes information on which herbs can be used against Ebola, and Epstein Barr.

Since modern medicine does not have a good treatment for viruses, I think exploring herbs that have been used for thousands of years is a good idea. If you keep these formulas handy and use them at the first sign of a cold, you might not even get a cold. How valuable would that be?

Constipation

There is only one point you need to know to treat constipation easily and effectively. That is Large Intestine 11. This point regulates and moistens the large intestine. Results are often achieved within five to ten minutes. Press very firmly on this point, as it can be a deep point, depending on how your arm is shaped. It is easy to grab the elbow and use your thumb on the point. You can treat one side or both sides. I would press on one side for five to ten minutes, then switch to the other side.

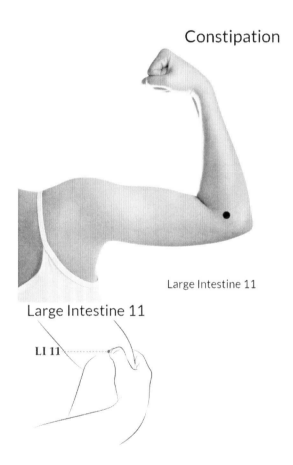

Constipation

Large Intestine 11

Large Intestine 11

LI 11

When I was in acupuncture school, over 20 years ago, people sometimes doubted if acupuncture actually worked at all. My answer was, let's treat Large Intestine 11, and Stomach 36 and see where we are in an hour. I used Stomach 36 to boost Large Intestine 11 to ensure success. I have not found this to be necessary, but it can also help regulate the intestines. To locate, put your fingers on your knee, where the top of the hand is on the eyes of the knee, the little indentations.

Constipation

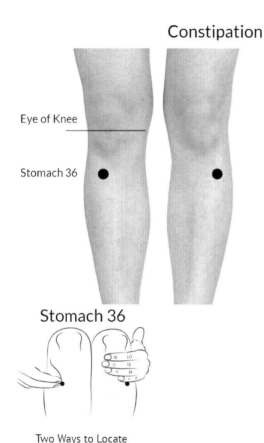

Eye of Knee

Stomach 36

Stomach 36

Two Ways to Locate

Treatment Notes

It is healthy to have at least one bowel movement every day. Some people believe that once a week is OK. People who have been constipated a long time can benefit from a colon cleanse. I like the Renew Life brand. Probiotics are very important for regularity. The bulk of your stool is bacteria. Garden of Life brand makes Primal Defense Ultra, which is a very good quality product.

Cough

There are different types of cough. If you have a cold or flu, your body is trying to get rid of the pathogen. Coughing from allergies can be treated by Large Intestine 4 and 11. This boosts your immune system and helps it to calm down. Large Intestine 11 also treats fever.

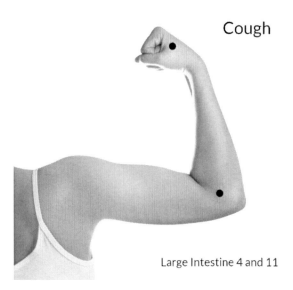

Cough

Large Intestine 4 and 11

Barking Cough
A Chinese medicine diagnosis of Lung phlegm heat would include the symptoms of a barking cough with profuse yellow mucus, fever, thirst, and chest oppression. This type of cough should send you to a medical doctor immediately, because it is often caused by an infection.

If the mucus is yellow, it usually means there is an infection, or it is on its way to becoming an infection that can turn into something that can kill you. When I say barking cough, that is a deep cough that sounds like the person is barking.

After you have seen your medical doctor, you can use acupressure to help yourself.

Lung 5, by the elbow, clears mucus and heat in the lungs, which is inflammation. This point is located on the thumb side of the arm, in the crook of the arm, by the biceps tendon. You can make a fist while locating the point and that makes it easy to find.

Cough

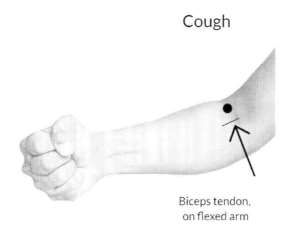

Biceps tendon,
on flexed arm

Lung 5

Stomach 40 is the phlegm point. It resolves excess mucus. It is located in the midpoint of the calf, two fingers from the shin bone. Since this is more difficult to locate, I will sometimes draw a circle around the point so I can treat it several times a day when someone is very sick. Stomach 36 strengthens the lungs and boosts the immune system.

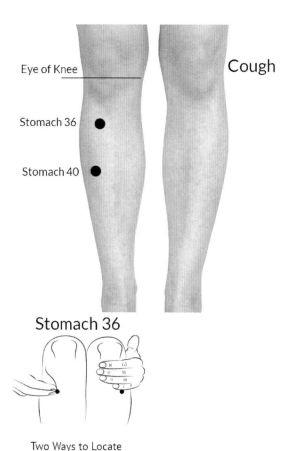

Two Ways to Locate

Weak Lungs Cough

A more common type of cough is caused by weak lungs. When you have a cold or flu or cough a lot, it weakens your lungs in Chinese medicine theory. If you have a slight cough with no mucus production, and fatigue, that is probably due to weak lung energy.

Lung 7 is often able to stop coughing pretty quickly. It is important to combine it with other points to treat the root cause of coughing.

Cough

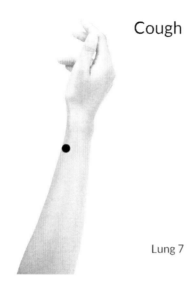

Lung 7

Lung 7 Location

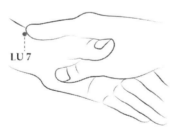

LU 7

Depression

There are many causes of depression. In Chinese medicine, it is not possible to be emotionally healthy if there is a physical health problem. There are numerous causes of depression, but my goal with this book is to offer information about the most common causes.

A common cause of depression is weak kidney energy. Giovanni Maciocia, who wrote many acupuncture textbooks, says that he treats the kidneys for all patients with depression, even if they do not present with kidney symptoms. Boosting the kidneys will provide more energy, and stress has a depleting effect on the adrenals as well.

Kidney 3 and 7 are my first choices to treat the kidneys. They are easy to locate, by the inner ankle bone. These points treat all aspects of the kidneys. They improve energy levels, and treat incontinence and other urinary issues.

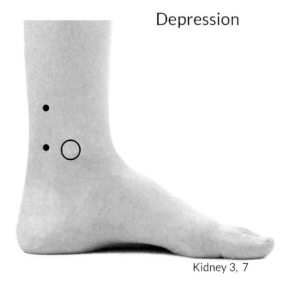

Depression

Kidney 3, 7

In Chinese medicine theory, our kidneys weaken as we age. This is a natural part of aging. That does not mean that we need to continue to suffer with this. It is easy to treat with Chinese medicine.

Chronic stress is a common cause of depression. This can be treated with Liver 3. This point is one of the most commonly used acupuncture points, because it regulates the liver which relieves stress, and improves digestion.

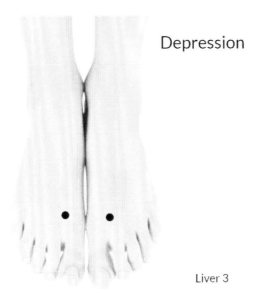

Depression

Liver 3

Boosting overall energy and digestion will improve all aspects of health. Stomach 36 boosts energy levels, improves digestion, and boosts the immune system. One of my teachers once said that people only need that point if they are a human being.

Depression

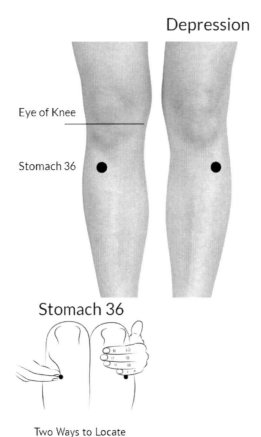

Eye of Knee

Stomach 36

Stomach 36

Two Ways to Locate

Treatment Notes

In addition to acupressure, I would consider taking kidney tonics like cordyceps. This is one of the most dependable herbs to boost energy levels quickly. There are two types of cordyceps supplements. One is the fruiting body, the other is the mycelium. With mushrooms there is a wide variation in quality. I have used mycelium products that were good, like Planetary Herbals, but other brands have not been so good.

The mycelium is essentially the new growth of the mushroom, so it is not mature. It has its own active constituents, but in my opinion the mature fruiting body is stronger. It is also the part most commonly used.

Krill oil can be helpful for depression. Our brain is made out of fat. If we do not have enough of the right kinds of fat, we cannot be mentally sharp.

Wheat is a common cause of depression. There are different theories as to why. Consider avoiding all grains for a while and see if that relieves your symptoms.

Thyroid issues can cause depression. There are literally dozens of things that can cause chronic depression. If you are not physically healthy, it is difficult to be emotionally healthy.

Your local licensed acupuncturist will be able to help you in many ways. It would not be difficult to write an entire book on how acupuncture and Chinese herbs can treat depression.

If you are interested in further study, Giovanni Maciocia wrote a book called *The Psyche in Chinese Medicine*. This book is an in depth analysis of different mental and emotional imbalances and how Chinese medicine can treat them successfully. There is always an answer in Chinese medicine. You just have to know where to look and not give up.

Diabetic Neuropathy

Diabetic neuropathy is nerve damage caused by high blood sugar, and or high insulin levels. The treatment is the same as any treatment in Chinese medicine. We need to restore healthy blood flow by stimulating the appropriate points. I have had great results using foot points with acupuncture.

I had a patient who had purple calves and feet. He could not walk without horrible pain. After 6 acupuncture sessions it no longer hurt to walk, and his feet and legs were pink again, which shows improved blood flow. Results will probably take longer with acupressure, but I believe acupressure would help.

When a body part is purple, that means the oxygen level is low. Some people would say the tissue is dead, but if it were dead, it would start rotting and turn black. Restoring circulation with acupuncture can improve tissue oxygen levels and prevent the need for surgery.

I would definitely get acupuncture as quickly as possible to reverse this condition, and follow up with acupressure between sessions. There is no time to waste with this problem. 80% of diabetic amputations begin with a foot ulcer. The open wound can easily get infected.

Every day about 230 Americans with diabetes will have an amputation. That is 83,950 per year! Please see your local acupuncturist as soon as you can for fast results.

The points used to treat foot neuropathy are located between the toes, and the strongest points on the leg. The idea is to treat multiple meridians on the foot and ankle. Any time you stimulate the acupuncture points, you are increasing circulation in that meridian, which will relieve pain and help heal the area. The most important points to treat are the points between the toes, Ba Feng, Stomach 41 on the top of the ankle, and the Stomach meridian. There are many options, but these are the ones I recommend and use.

The spleen meridian on the foot is located below the foot bones. You will be able to feel the foot bones when you massage them. Since the points are located using the bones, the flesh image makes it a bit harder to find the points on the image. Just press your foot and massage just below the toe and foot bones. That is where the points are located. You do not need to be exact with your location, massage multiple points in that area with a mini massager, but not directly on an open wound.

Diabetic Neuropathy

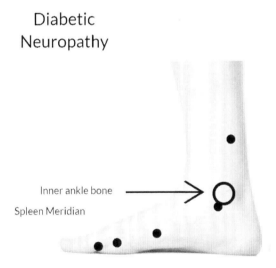

Inner ankle bone

Spleen Meridian

If you have an open wound, you should see your local acupuncturist to do what is called a "surround the dragon" treatment. That is where tiny needles are placed around the wound, which improves blood flow. The lack of circulation is what causes the wound to not close, so improving circulation in that area will speed healing.

Daily treatment with acupressure could be very helpful to improve blood flow.

The Ba Feng points are used to strongly pull circulation into the toes. Treating the end of the foot is a strong way to improve blood flow all the way down the leg.

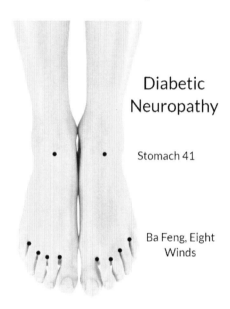

Diabetic
Neuropathy

Stomach 41

Ba Feng, Eight
Winds

Stomach 36 is one of the most commonly used acupuncture points. In addition to hundreds of other functions, it improves blood flow in the leg. Spleen 6 helps to improve wound healing anywhere on the body. Stomach 41 is on top of the foot, it is a key point to treat drop foot, or any foot pain or circulation problem. I would treat Stomach 36, 40, and 41 daily. The Stomach meridian is the strongest meridian on the leg to treat leg and foot disorders.

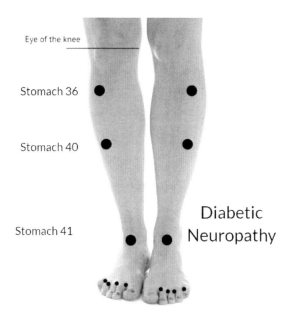

Eye of the knee

Stomach 36

Stomach 40

Stomach 41

Diabetic
Neuropathy

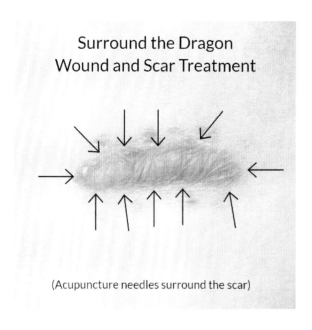

Surround the Dragon
Wound and Scar Treatment

(Acupuncture needles surround the scar)

Treatment Notes

Acupuncture alone is enough to restore circulation in the feet and legs. I have not used acupressure alone, but I believe it would help. Anything that you do that improves blood flow or increases circulation will help. Since I cannot know your personal condition, please consult your doctor before you try treating yourself. Please do not accept the inevitability of amputation. With the right care, you might recover faster than you think.

Diarrhea

There are several types of diarrhea. If you ate something bad, diarrhea is not a bad thing. Your body needs to get rid of what you ate. Chronic diarrhea can have several causes. Digestive weakness is the most common. There are several acupressure points that treat diarrhea effectively.

Stomach 25 is the first point to try. This point is about two finger widths away from the belly button. It treats about 20 things including constipation, diarrhea, colitis, and intestinal obstruction. It works by regulating the intestines.

Diarrhea

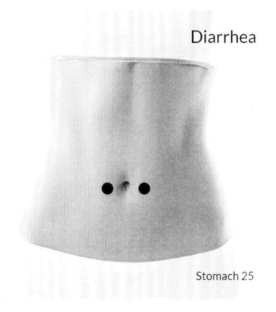

Stomach 25

Chronic diarrhea is often caused by weak digestion. The best points to treat that are Stomach 36 and 37. Stomach 36 looks hard to find, but once you know how to measure, it is easy. The size of the point is fairly large, so don't worry too much about missing it. It is one of the strongest and most important acupuncture points. Please refer to my book,

Acupuncture Points Handbook, for the dozens of functions and indications of this point.

If in doubt on which point to treat, choose Stomach 36, it is that strong. It is used to strengthen the immune system and digestion, regulate the stomach and intestines, treat diaphragm spasms, fatigue, asthma, colds and flu, the list is endless.

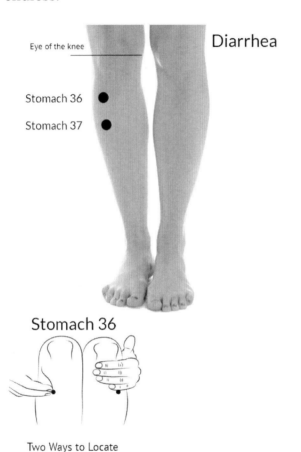

All you need to do is place your hand on your knee. The point is located just below your little finger, about an inch from the shin bone.

Stomach 37 is located one hand width, or 3 cun, below Stomach 36. It treats diarrhea, gastritis, leg pain and atrophy, intestinal inflammation, and many other things.

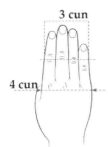

Treatment Notes

Ginger root is very effective to treat diarrhea. I like Jarrow ginger root extract, it comes in capsules, so you do not have to take as many pills. A lack of beneficial gut bacteria can be at the root of diarrhea and any intestinal problem. There are several great products including the Jarrow acidophilus, and Garden of Life Primal Defense, which is a homeostatic soil organism, or HSO. These bacteria used to be on fresh produce, which was how most people got their gut bacteria. A great book on this issue is called *Eat Dirt*, by Dr. Josh Axe. He explains how to restore intestinal health.

Dizziness

I was hesitant to write a chapter on dizziness, because so many things can cause dizziness. There are dozens of possibilities. High blood pressure can cause it, so if you are dizzy you should always be evaluated by your medical doctor, and please check your blood pressure regularly.

Although, there can be many causes of dizziness, there are also some common causes that you can easily treat yourself.

Sinus inflammation can cause dizziness. The sinuses become inflamed and swollen, which can put pressure on the nerves in your ear, causing dizziness. For quick relief of sinus pain, you can treat points that open the sinuses. You won't know which part of your sinuses are inflamed, so it is easier to treat all three points.

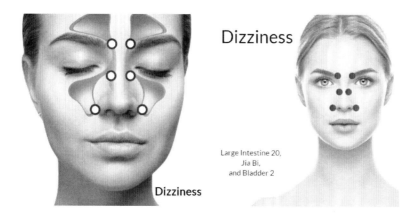

Dizziness

Large Intestine 20,
Jia Bi,
and Bladder 2

Dizziness

If dizziness is caused by a queasy stomach, Pericardium 6 is a good point to use. It regulates the heart and stomach to relieve digestive and other chest problems. It is located on a flat hand, 2 cun from the wrist crease.

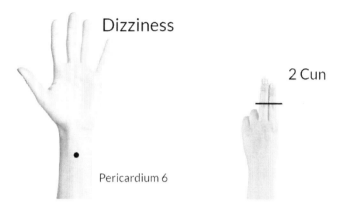

If ear problems are causing dizziness, Small Intestine 19 helps restore healthy ear circulation. It treats ear discharge, ear inflammation, tinnitus, and vertigo that is caused by ear problems.

Gallbladder 2 is just below Small Intestine 19. It restores healthy circulation in the ears to treat hearing loss, jaw pain, and ear infections. Ear infections are often caused by a virus, so antiviral herbs like Andrographis can be used to treat the virus. Gallbladder 2 and Small Intestine 19 are very sensitive areas, so if you treat them, be very gentle.

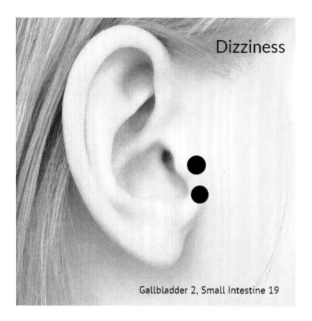

Dizziness

Gallbladder 2, Small Intestine 19

A common cause of dizziness is tight muscles at the base of the skull. When the muscles are tight, they put pressure on the nerves and blood vessels that lead to the ear.

One of my patients was using an inversion table. These tables are marketed to treat back pain. One day he became very dizzy and had vertigo. The room was spinning for him and he threw up due to the nausea.

He had not been dizzy before, but when he hung nearly upside down on the table, this put extra pressure on the vertebrae in his neck. I believe he had a pre-existing problem in that area, and when he put too much pressure on it, it caused a compression of the tissue in the area, which caused the joint to be slightly off where it was supposed to be. He also said that he heard a sound when he turned his head side to side. I believe that the discs in his neck are worn down, and that is what is causing the noise.

The image below shows the Gallbladder 20 point, and the circles represent the area to treat. This is where the neck muscles attach to the head. Be very gentle in this area!

134

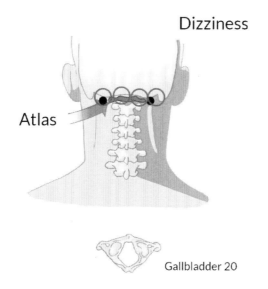

Dizziness

Atlas

Gallbladder 20

The bones in your body fit together like pieces of a puzzle. If you make sudden movements you can cause a slight misalignment of the bones and joints, as well as irritating the nerves when the muscles tighten up.

I treated the points at the base of his skull, and in his upper neck. After one treatment his dizziness went away.

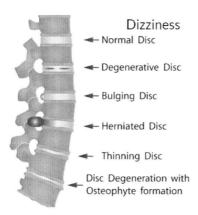

Dizziness
← Normal Disc
← Degenerative Disc
← Bulging Disc
← Herniated Disc
← Thinning Disc
Disc Degeneration with Osteophyte formation

I had personally experienced this myself. When I first graduated from acupuncture school I was subleasing space from a chiropractor. I was curious to find out what type of treatments he did, so I let him use an activator on my back and neck. Afterwards, I was dizzy for three weeks.

I finally realized this was not going away on its own, and it must have been caused by damage done by the activator. He was very aggressive with this device, and I think it is a bit nuts to hit people hard at the base of the skull. The bones, nerves, blood vessels, and joint tissue in this area are very sensitive.

I took matters into my own hands and inserted needles at the base of the skull, at the hairline at the back of the head. Afterwards the dizziness went away.

My cousin called me once to tell me his wife was dizzy. She had been on a rollercoaster ride and had been dizzy ever since. I suggested that her neck was slightly off in the area of the atlas. She could try gentle massage in that area to relax the muscles and allow the joint to go back in place. It worked for her.

Gently press on the sore areas at the base of your head. When you feel soreness, you know it is probably inflamed and needs attention. I would gently press in that entire area. Consider 5-10 minutes per spot.

Gallstones can also cause dizziness and nausea, please refer to that chapter for more information.

Ear Pain

Ear pain is caused by a blockage of circulation in the ear. As with any type of pain, you can treat the meridians that affect the ear, as well as other points that can restore circulation there.

Triple Warmer 17 is located behind the earlobe. It relieves ear pain, treats itching inside the ear, redness, pain and swelling of the ear. It also treats lockjaw. Redness, pain and swelling can be caused by an ear infection and your medical doctor should be consulted. The ears can be damaged by untreated infections.

Triple Warmer 21 is located in the slight depression at the root of the top of the ear. It treats earache by opening and regulating the ears. It restores normal circulation in the ears.

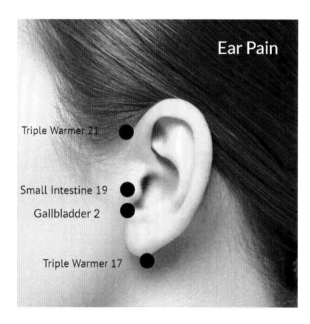

Small Intestine 19 is located right in front of the ear. It is easier to locate as a small hole if the mouth is open, but you do not need to do that. Just treat the area. This point strongly improves circulation in the ear to treat many disorders. In Chinese medicine theory pain is caused by a lack of circulation in the painful area. When you restore healthy blood flow the pain goes away. Small Intestine 19 treats tinnitus, ear inflammation, and headache due to ear issues.

Gallbladder 2 is right in front of the ear. It opens the ears to treat deafness, tinnitus, ear pain, jaw pain, hearing loss and TMJ pain. In Chinese medicine the expression that a point "opens" means that it strongly opens the meridian to improve blood flow and restore function. Although this point is listed as treating tinnitus, there are many causes of tinnitus and Chinese herbal medicine is often necessary.

Large Intestine 4 is used to treat any pain on the head. It restores healthy circulation to the ear. Large Intestine treats fevers, colds, and flu. Large Intestine 4 is the more important of these two points for ear pain, but if there is an infection or inflammation, Large Intestine 11 is nice to use. These points also treat allergies and sinus issues.

Ear Pain

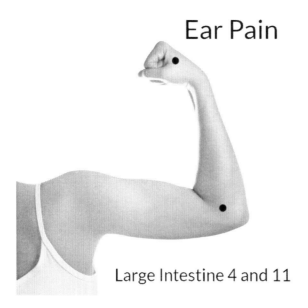

Large Intestine 4 and 11

Ear pain can also be caused by sinus and allergies. Please see refer to those chapters for the points.

Treatment Notes

There are oils formulated to treat ear pain and infections. Wally's Ear Oil is a famous product and includes garlic and other antibacterial, and antiviral herbs to be used topically.

Elbow Pain

To relieve elbow pain, the first choice is the Large Intestine meridian. That is the meridian on the arm that is the strongest to treat any type of pain on the arm.

Large Intestine 4 and 11 are used as the strongest points to activate the meridian and relieve pain.

Quyangwei is an extra point that Giovanni Maciocia referenced in his books. It is located next to the epicondyle, which is next to Large Intestine 11.

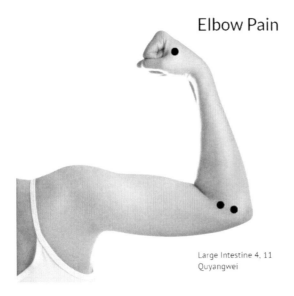

Elbow Pain

Large Intestine 4, 11
Quyangwei

Treatment Notes
Elbow pain is often caused by tendinitis. I like FYI Restore enzymes from Garden of Life, or bromelain for this. It resolves the inflammation quickly. The enzymes can be taken on an empty stomach as needed.

Eye Pain

Eye pain is sometimes caused by sinus blockage. Pain anywhere on the face can be caused by sinus blockage or inflammation. Please have your eyes checked if you have any type of eye pain. My mom had a detached retina and she thought it was sinus pain. You cannot take chances with your eyes.

Acupuncture cannot treat a detached retina, you need surgery for that. After her surgery I did acupuncture with tiny needles around her opposite eye to speed healing. Please check out the chapter on Lasik dry eyes. This is a serious problem and there are acupuncture solutions.

The best points for sinus blockage are located on the nose. In my experience, these work the fastest and they are easy to use. The reason that sinus problems can cause eye pain is that the swelling puts pressure nerves and blood vessels on the face.

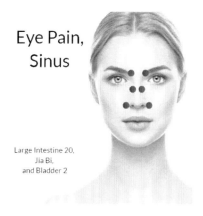

Eye Pain, Sinus

Large Intestine 20,
Jia Bi,
and Bladder 2

Many eye diseases can be treated with acupuncture and Chinese herbs. As we age, our hormones decline, this can cause tissue weakness and dryness.

Acupuncture restores healthy blood flow, which can strengthen tissue that is deprived of healthy circulation, as well as regulate the nerves that affect the eyes. I know it seems unbelievable that acupuncture can treat eye diseases, but many people have gotten treatment with acupuncture and a new system of micro-acupuncture, which uses points on the hands and feet. Do not give up. There is almost always a way to improve eye diseases with Chinese medicine.

Any problem on the face can be treated with Large Intestine 4.

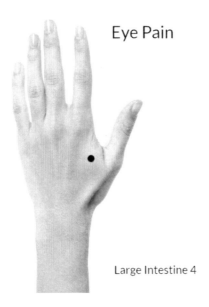

Eye Pain

Large Intestine 4

Fatigue

Acupuncture and Chinese herbs excel at relieving fatigue. Most patients report feeling better than they have in years after just one month of acupuncture. Very often we decline in energy levels and do not even remember what it felt like to have good energy levels.

The most common causes of fatigue are a weakness in the kidney energy, and digestive weakness and irregularity.

Even if you do not have obvious symptoms of a kidney deficiency, it will boost energy to treat the kidneys.

The most common symptoms of a kidney weakness are:

Kidney Yin Deficiency
- Night sweats
- Hot flashes
- Dizziness
- Thirst
- Sore back
- Tinnitus
- Deafness
- Ache in the bones
- Hot palms and soles of the feet
- Poor memory
- Dry mouth at night

Kidney Yang Deficiency
- Abundant, clear urination
- Apathy
- Aversion to cold
- Edema of the legs
- Impotence

- Infertility in women
- Premature ejaculation
- Back pain
- Weak knees
- Weak legs
- Waking at night to urinate
- Incontinence

You might notice that a kidney yin deficiency corresponds to a lot of problems women have in menopause and perimenopause. Chinese herbs are very helpful to treat all aspects of kidney weakness, including hot flashes. There are numerous formulas that treat the root cause of these symptoms for lasting relief.

Treating the kidney points will treat all aspects of kidney weakness, which treats fatigue caused by kidney weakness.

Please remember that a diagnosis of a kidney deficiency in Chinese medicine has no correlation to a Western medicine diagnosis. Your kidney organs are probably fine. This is Chinese medicine. It is a completely different way of diagnosing and treating disease, which has been used effectively for thousands of years.

To treat fatigue caused by kidney weakness, the points Kidney 3, 6, and 7 are the best choices. I have even used these points to treat patients on kidney dialysis, so do not doubt how strong they are. One of my patients had kidney damage, which she suspected was a result of an antibiotic she took. We were able to improve kidney function and avoid dialysis by doing acupuncture twice a week for a few weeks.

To locate the points, you need to locate the ankle bone on the inside of the leg. This bone is a little rounded area that is called a medial malleolus. This bone is large in some people, and in some people it is small and not as easy to see, but you can feel the bone if you press.

I am including an image from my point location book, because a line drawing clearly shows where the points are in relation to the inner ankle bone. A flesh image of Kidney 3, 6, and 7 is below that. Kidney 7 is 2 cun above Kidney 3.

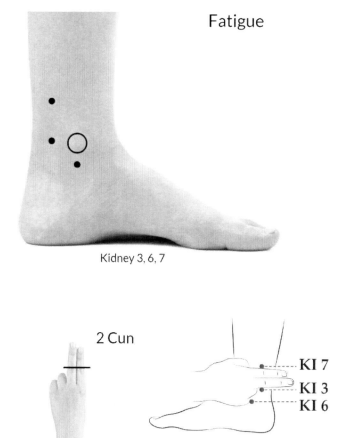

Fatigue

Kidney 3, 6, 7

2 Cun

KI 7
KI 3
KI 6

Kidney 3 is the most important point to treat. It is located just behind the inner ankle bone. It treats fatigue, frequent urination, heel pain, incontinence, insomnia, and urgent urination. If you treat only one kidney point, this is the one to use.

Kidney 7 is used to treat incontinence, nephritis, foot pain, and to regulate urination, among other things.

Kidney 6 is located about one finger width below the inner ankle bone. It is used to treat kidney disorders, hot flashes, insomnia, sore throat, uterine prolapse, and it also can help to expedite labor. This point is very calming and can be used for anxiety and insomnia. I would not use it on a woman who might be or is pregnant. It pulls energy down from the head, so it has a descending action. That is one reason it is so great for anxiety. Soaking your feet in warm water has the same effect. It pulls energy down, away from the head.

Another common cause of fatigue is digestive weakness. If you cannot digest your food well, you cannot have good energy levels. In Chinese medicine, we always ask questions about digestion and energy levels. In order to be healthy and pain free, you will need improved energy levels and digestion. In most cases we can treat all of your ailments at the same time. If you have pain, we can treat that at the same time as we treat fatigue, insomnia, and other problems. That is why it is such a holistic treatment. You are treated head to toe.

The best point to improve digestion is Stomach 36. This is probably the most important acupuncture point. It has so many functions, and everyone can benefit from better energy levels.

The most common symptoms of a digestive weakness, or Spleen energy deficiency in Chinese medicine, are:

- Poor appetite

- Nausea
- Digestive issues
- Eating disorders
- Loose stools
- Undigested food in stool
- Dull stomach pain
- Easily sweating without exertion
- Gas and abdominal distension
- Tiredness or weakness
- Difficulty waking in the morning
- Weak muscles
- Dull achy pain in muscles
- Easy bruising
- Obsessive worry or obsessive thoughts

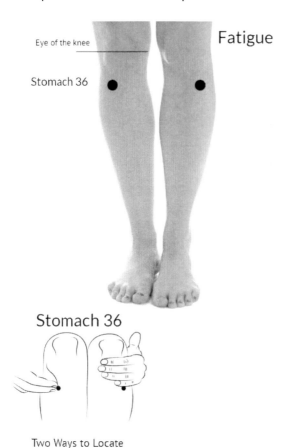

Eye of the knee

Stomach 36

Fatigue

Stomach 36

Two Ways to Locate

Treatment Notes

Improving digestion and energy levels is a part of every acupuncture treatment. In addition to acupuncture and Chinese herbs, many other things can cause fatigue. To list a few, candida, Epstein Barr virus, adrenal fatigue, and food intolerances. At the bare minimum, consider taking a good multivitamin to ensure you have enough of the vitamins your body needs to make energy. I like the Garden of Life brand Raw Vitamins. They make a one a day product also.

Fever

Fever can be a very serious issue. Normal body temperature is around 98.6. Delirium and convulsions can result from high body temperatures. A temperature of 104 degrees is commonly held to be dangerous, although anything over 100 should be checked out by a medical doctor.

Large Intestine 11 is the number one point to use to reduce fevers. This point is also used to boost the immune system to treat colds and flu, and allergies.

I once had a patient in her seventies who had the flu. She refused to see a medical doctor. She kept calling me, telling me her mother was trying to speak to her through her clock radio. I finally went to her house to try to convince her to go to the hospital. She was bright red and had a fever. She appeared to be dehydrated. I treated Large Intestine 11, and her body cooled off in about an hour. She was finally convinced to go to the hospital. Since she had had a fever for a while, she was dehydrated and needed intravenous fluids to replenish her body. Always take a fever seriously.

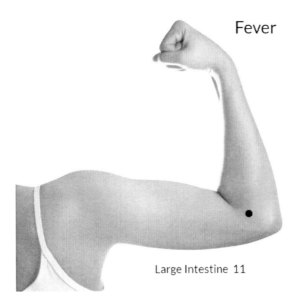

Fever

Large Intestine 11

After treating Large Intestine 11 for the fever, I would consider treating Stomach 36 to boost the immune system. There are additional points in the cold and flu section.

Fever

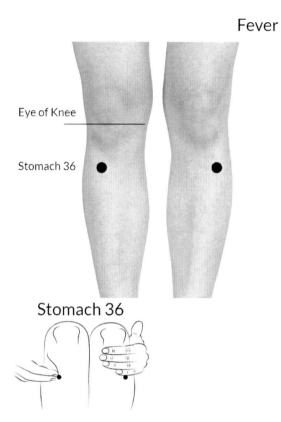

Eye of Knee

Stomach 36

Stomach 36

Two Ways to Locate

151

Finger Pain

Any type of finger pain can be relieved with Ba Xie points. The translation is Eight Pathogens. It is pronounced "Bah Shay." The points are located between the fingers. Acupressure will be easier to do if you form a fist with your hand, it enlarges the space between the fingers. Stimulating these points increases circulation all the way down the arm. These points treat any type of hand pain or stiffness.

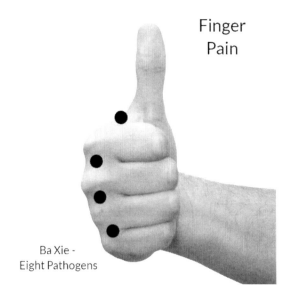

Finger
Pain

Ba Xie -
Eight Pathogens

If you have thumb pain, Large Intestine 4 can be used in addition to Eight Pathogens.

Finger Pain

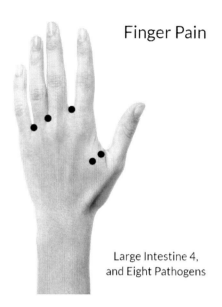

Large Intestine 4,
and Eight Pathogens

Foot Pain

Foot pain can be caused by an injury. It can also be caused by excess fluid building up in the legs and feet. This puts pressure on the nerves in the feet.

A set of acupuncture points that is called Eight Winds, or Ba Feng, is very helpful to relieve foot and toe pain. These are the points I use to treat diabetic neuropathy. They strongly stimulate healthy blood flow to the feet. They can be used for any type of foot pain. If your feet are very swollen, you will need to reduce excess fluid before these will work as well.

Swelling or Edema

If you press firmly on your foot for a minute or two and there is an indentation remaining when you remove your finger, you have edema or swelling. This type of foot pain needs to be addressed by stimulating the body to get rid of fluids. Edema is tissue swelling caused by your body retaining excess fluid. If you have this problem, I suggest you get acupuncture and herbs, because this can be a serious problem. I will include the points for edema.

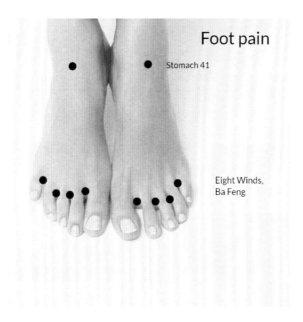

Another point that treats foot pain is Stomach 41. This is located at the level of the ankle, in the depression between the tendons on the top of the foot. This point is amazing. It treats ankle pain, foot drop, and lower leg pain and stiffness.

To relieve foot swelling, the best choice is Spleen 9. This point is used to relieve excess fluid in the body. Please refer to the water retention section for more points to treat this.

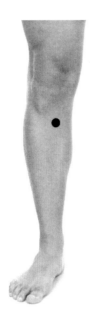

Foot Pain

Spleen 9

Frequent Urination, Weak Bladder, Incontinence

The most common cause for urinary weakness is weak kidney energy. In Chinese medicine theory, as we age, our kidney energy declines. Our kidneys are responsible for bladder control, as well as stool control. If the kidneys are very weak, the bladder is too weak to hold the urine, and the body cannot hold the stool. There is no reason to suffer from this. It is very treatable with Chinese medicine.

In addition to acupuncture and acupressure, there are Chinese herbal formulas that quickly improve your kidneys, and restore bladder control. It is possible to prevent and treat the root cause of incontinence, which can force people to use incontinence pads or adult diapers. I treat this very often in men and women. They are always surprised they improve so quickly.

The most important points to treat incontinence are Kidney 3, 6, and 7. This is a strong treatment to resolve kidney issues.

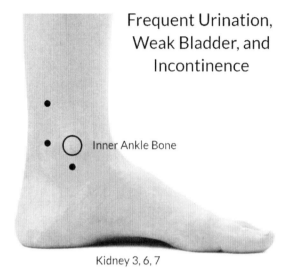

Frequent Urination, Weak Bladder, and Incontinence

Inner Ankle Bone

Kidney 3, 6, 7

Treatment Notes

There is a long history in Chinese medicine of using kidney tonic herbs to treat the symptoms of aging, such as osteoarthritis, pain, and urinary weakness. The herbs can also be used to boost energy levels and improve quality of life.

Cordyceps is an example of a Chinese herb that strengthens the kidneys. Your licensed acupuncturist will prescribe strong herbs to restore your kidneys quickly. Taking kidney tonic herbs is one of the most rejuvenating things you can do for your health, but there is no faster way to mess yourself up than to take kidney herbs that are not right for you.

The side effects of taking kidney herbs that are not appropriate for you are hot flashes, insomnia, and facial hair in women. Your licensed acupuncturist will have training in Chinese herbs for a quick resolution of this problem.

Gallstones

Many people have their gallbladders removed due to gallstones. I believe this should be the last option. There are many ways to treat them naturally.

The symptoms of gallstones include nausea, vomiting, sweating, fever, and chills. If the bile is blocked, you might have clay colored stools. You might also have back and shoulder pain.

There is a special acupuncture point specifically to treat gallstones. I am including the point next to it, Gallbladder 34, which can be used to regulate the gallbladder and liver. I have used the gallstone point once and it was very effective. I know this is a bit difficult to locate, but I wanted to include it in this book.

The Gallbladder Point, Dan Nang Xue, is located below the knee, on the side of the lower leg. In Chinese medicine terms, it clears gallbladder heat, or inflammation. It is located 1-2 cun below Gallbladder 34. Gallbladder 34 is below and in front of the head of the fibula bone, which is next to the shin bone.

Gallstones

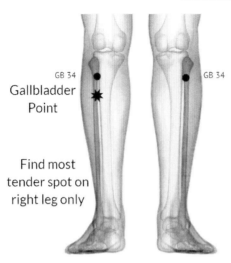

GB 34
Gallbladder
Point

GB 34

Find most
tender spot on
right leg only

Treatment Notes

There are numerous herbs that have been used for centuries to dissolve stones. Planetary Herbals makes a great product that contains herbs for gallstones and kidney stones called Stone Free. Always consult your doctor. Gallstones can cause serious problems.

Apple juice also dissolves gallstones. The husband of one of my patients had gallstones and he refused to take herbs for them. She learned that apple juice would dissolve them, so she simply gave him apple juice every day until they dissolved. It appears that the malic acid in the apples dissolves the stones.

Hand Pain

Hand pain can be caused by an injury of the hand, such as a repetitive stress injury from typing all day, or jamming your finger in a door. Any finger or hand pain can be treated by using these points. They restore healthy circulation to the hands, which will relieve pain. These points are located in the webs between the fingers. They are easier to access when you make a fist.

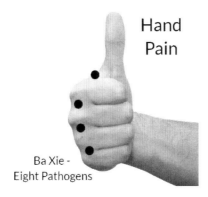

Hand
Pain

Ba Xie -
Eight Pathogens

Large Intestine 4 can be combined with Large Intestine 11, to activate the strongest meridian on the arm, the Large Intestine meridian. These points are often used together to treat arm pain.

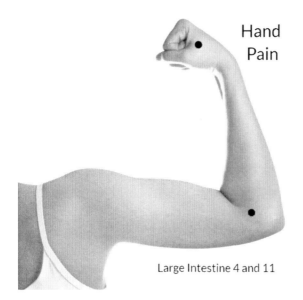

Hand
Pain

Large Intestine 4 and 11

Headache

There are many causes of headaches, including allergies, sinusitis, colds and flu, and stress. Please refer to the chapter on migraines, because there are additional points for migraines.

The first point to use to treat any type of headache is Large Intestine 4. This point treats allergies, cold and flu, ear infections, nosebleed, sinus congestion, toothache, and any problem on the face. It is known as the "face point." This point is famous for treating headaches.

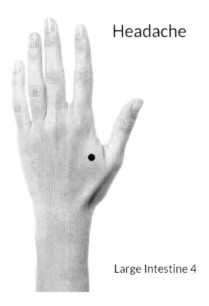

Headache

Large Intestine 4

I would treat this point for 10 minutes on each side and see if the headache goes away. Then move on to the next points. Acupressure, like acupuncture, is actually a diagnostic tool. Treating points helps you to determine the root cause by ruling things out.

A common cause of headaches is sinus inflammation, or sinusitis. Large Intestine 4 does treat sinus headaches, but if that does not solve the problem, I would try the sinus points next.

The first point to try is Jia Bi. This point is a good choice for acupressure. It is located just below the nasal bone. You can often feel relief within minutes. It is pronounced "Jaw Bee."

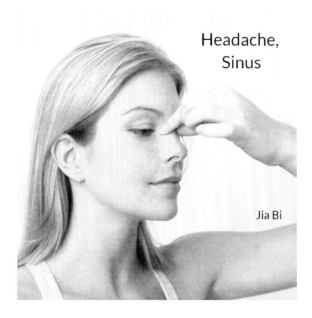

Headache,
Sinus

Jia Bi

Please refer to the sinus section for more sinus points.

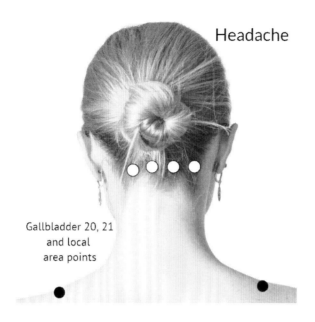

Headache

Gallbladder 20, 21
and local
area points

Some headaches are caused by tight neck and shoulder muscles. Firm but gentle pressure on Gallbladder 20 can help release the neck muscles. Gallbladder 21 is at the top of the shoulders. Massage in that area to help release the neck muscles. Massage at the back of the hairline, which is where many muscles attach. Press firmly to relax the muscles.

One of my favorite ways to treat neck pain is by using ear seeds for acupressure. These points are easy to locate and very effective to relieve tight neck muscles and any type of neck pain. Stress often causes tense muscles. The traditional way to treat these points is Vaccaria seeds. This is a black seed that is attached to tiny piece of tape. Simply apply the seed to the area of your ear that treats the neck. I usually use about 4 ear seeds to cover the whole area. Press on the seed several times a day and as needed.

The ear is a microcosm of the body. That means that your entire body is mapped on your ear. All areas of your body, and all internal organs are represented on the ear. I especially like treating back and neck issues via the ear.

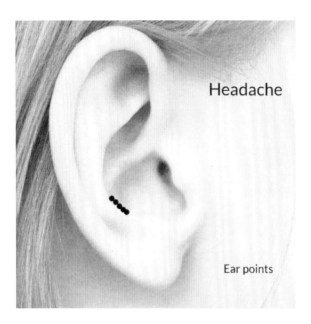

Headache

Ear points

The seeds will naturally fall off after you wash your hair a couple of times. Treat one side for a couple of days, then switch to the other ear, giving the first ear you treated a rest from treatment.

Heart Arrhythmia

This section is called heart arrhythmia, but Chinese medicine would consider it a heart imbalance and the diagnosis would be made via the pulse. In modern times these points have been shown to regulate the heart.

Points on the heart meridian regulate the heart energy. Heart 7 is very commonly used for anxiety. Any emotion in excess can affect the heart, which grows weaker and can cause things like anxiety, and insomnia. It is easy to treat this point with either a mini massager, or using your fingertip.

Heart 5 is the primary point to use for an irregular heartbeat. Heart 5 and 7 can be combined in the same treatment. You can use your thumbnail to treat these points.

Pericardium 6 can be used to open the circulation in the chest. This helps treat stomach issues also. It is located while holding the hand flat, do not bend back the hand. It is 2 cun from the wrist crease.

Heart Arrhythmia

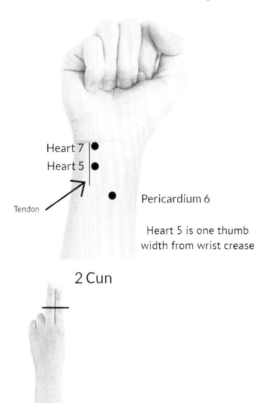

Heart 7

Heart 5

Pericardium 6

Tendon

Heart 5 is one thumb width from wrist crease

2 Cun

Heart 7

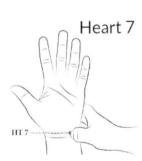

HT 7

Obviously, this is a very serious matter and you should always consult your doctor if you believe you have an issue. Chinese medicine treats health problems on an energetic level. Sometimes Western testing is done that does not reveal an imbalance. Chinese medicine excels at treating problems on an energetic level, before they are seen as a problem by Western medicine.

Treatment Notes

Many herbs are used in Chinese medicine to restore chest circulation. There are herbs that strengthen the heart, regulate blood flow in the heart, and calm it down when a heart imbalance is causing insomnia or anxiety.

Sometimes it is hard to tell if something is related to the heart or the stomach. Any constriction in that area can make you feel it is your heart, when it is your stomach. I have seen hiatal hernias cause similar symptoms to a heart attack. Please consult with your local emergency room if you have any doubts whatsoever.

One of the most popular herbal heart tonics is hawthorn berry. It is a gentle tonic and it has been used in Europe for many years to treat heart problems. In Chinese medicine hawthorn berry is used to improve the digestion of fats.

Hawthorn berry is used in candy in China, in the same way that cherry is used in the West. It has a nice flavor. You can buy the hawthorn berry extract powder and make it into a tea. It is called Shan Zha in Chinese, and herbal extracts come in 100 gram bottles. If you prefer to take capsules, Planetary Herbals has a good hawthorn extract product in capsules. This product might reduce your blood pressure and reduce the thickness of your blood. If you are being treated by a physician, I would always ask them if it is OK for you.

Hiccups

The first point to try to treat hiccups is Ren 12, because it regulates the esophagus. Ren 12 is located one hand width above the belly button, on the midline. It regulates the stomach, treats acid reflux, and treats gastritis. Ren 13 regulates the stomach, and Ren 14 regulates the diaphragm. Ren 12 is located one hand width above the belly button. Ren 13 is one cun or thumb width above Ren 12, and Ren 14 is one cun above Ren 13.

Hiccups

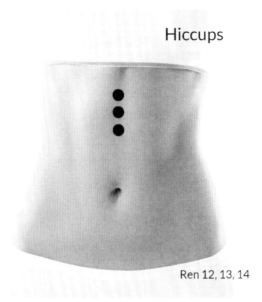

Ren 12, 13, 14

Pericardium 6 is on the wrist, two fingers away from the wrist crease, in the middle. This point regulates the stomach and relieves blocked circulation in the chest.

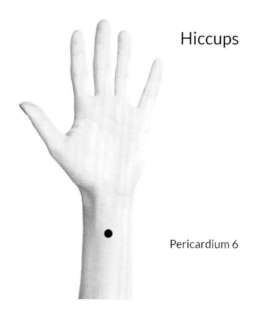

Hiccups

Pericardium 6

Liver 3 is used to regulate the liver and treat stress. Sometimes stress can cause hiccups. It does this by invading the stomach. I know that sounds nuts, but energetically when the liver energy is not circulating properly, it can affect the stomach in Chinese medicine theory.

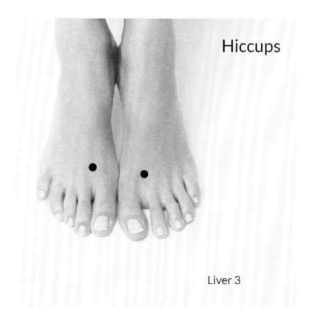

Hiccups

Liver 3

171

The symptoms that would help you determine if the liver is at the root cause of hiccups are reflux, irritability, belching, burning in the stomach, slight pain above the stomach, nausea, and vomiting.

Some people actually become nauseated when they get stressed out. In Chinese medicine theory, the liver energy can invade the stomach energy. I once had a patient who became nauseated every morning before work. Thinking about going to work stressed her out, which caused her symptoms.

Stress can also cause the liver to invade the spleen, which can cause diarrhea. Pay attention to your symptoms and notate if symptoms start at a certain time of the day, such as getting ready for a stressful job, or dealing with someone who frustrates you. Liver 3 will help relieve this.

Treatment Notes
Hiccups can be treated by the old standby of drinking a glass of water. This helps to encourage the muscles in the esophagus to regulate themselves.

High Blood Pressure

In Chinese medicine theory, high blood pressure is usually caused by a liver imbalance, or a kidney weakness. There is a deficiency of liver yin, which causes the yang to rise. I know that sounds crazy, but that is how it is explained. There are other causes, but that is the most common one.

Since every person is different, you cannot just use the same acupuncture points on everyone and get good results. A full diagnosis is made, and the kidneys, and liver and any other organ that is out of balance is treated. However, there are several points that are most commonly used to lower blood pressure. I believe that the modern causes of high blood pressure are often not the same as what might have caused the symptoms of high blood pressure in ancient China.

There seems to be about a fifty percent chance of success using these points, and it will not hurt. As with all acupuncture points, they regulate the body.

High
Blood
Pressure

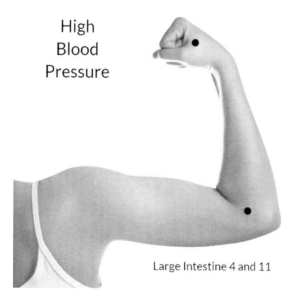

Large Intestine 4 and 11

Large intestine 4 and 11 balance the body.

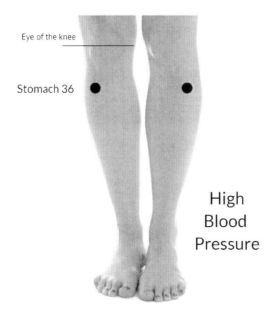

Eye of the knee

Stomach 36

High
Blood
Pressure

Since the liver is the root of many problems, it is important to treat the liver. Large intestine 4 is often combined with Liver 3 to balance the energy in the body. It is called Four Gates. It balances the upper body with the lower body. Stomach 36 boosts digestion, the immune system and improves energy. Liver 3 is the number one point to use for stress.

Most research on acupuncture for blood pressure includes these points. I do not think it is a magic bullet. The Chinese medicine theory of a lack of liver yin causing high blood pressure could be correlated with the modern clogged liver. When the blood is thicker, the heart has to pump harder, which can raise pressure.

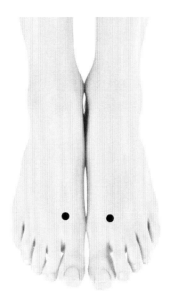

High
Blood
Pressure

Liver 3

Most people do not want to change their diet, so I suggest they see a medical doctor and take medications to treat high blood pressure. This is not a disease you want to ignore. Checking your blood pressure regularly is important. Your doctor will tell you what is best for you.

If you are already on medication for blood pressure, you will need to carefully monitor it daily if you start acupressure and supplements. If your blood pressure goes too low, you could pass out, or become very tired.

Treatment Notes
Hawthorn berry is used to gently strengthen and regulate the heart. Planetary Herbals makes a good product in capsules. Hawthorn berry is drunk as a tea in China. If you want to try hawthorn berry extract in tea form, look for the name Shan Zha. That is the Chinese name. It has a great flavor, but you will need to add a little sweetener, because it is slightly sour.

CoQ10 is a premiere heart tonic. Statin drugs deplete CoQ10. I believe anyone over 40 should consider taking CoQ10. Dosages of 400 to 600 milligrams have been used to treat heart failure. The technical name for CoQ10 is Ubiquinone.

There is a newer and more effective form of CoQ10 called Ubiquinol. It is better absorbed in people over age 40. Jarrow makes an excellent product. I have heard of someone who started taking CoQ10 and he had to reduce his dosage, because it lowered his blood pressure too much, because he was already on medications. Please consult your doctor if you want to try anything in this section.

Hives

Hives are itchy red areas on the skin. They are most commonly caused by an allergic reaction.

Large Intestine 4 and 11 are used to boost the immune system to treat any type of allergic response. Allergies are typically caused by a weak immune system overreacting to things it would not normally respond to if the immune system were healthy.

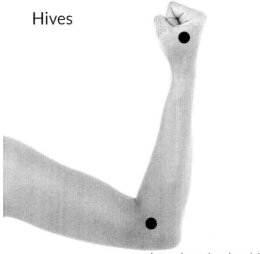

Hives

Large Intestine 4 and 11

Spleen 10 is used to regulate the blood and clear heat. That can correlate to inflammation. This point can be used to treat all skin disorders caused by inflammation, as well as itching anywhere in the body. Spleen 10 is also used in combination with other points to treat knee pain. It is located two finger widths above the kneecap.

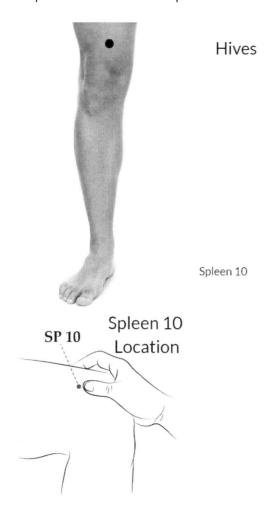

Hives

Spleen 10

SP 10   Spleen 10
         Location

Spleen 6 treats skin diseases, regulates hormones, treats edema, and anxiety. Although an allergic reaction is the cause of hives, there are often underlying health issues that can contribute. Spleen 6 treats the blood, which is a Chinese medicine concept that cannot be defined easily using Western medicine theory. Anemia can sometimes be correlated to a blood deficiency. Chinese medicine treats blood weakness and imbalance before Western medicine is able to detect it.

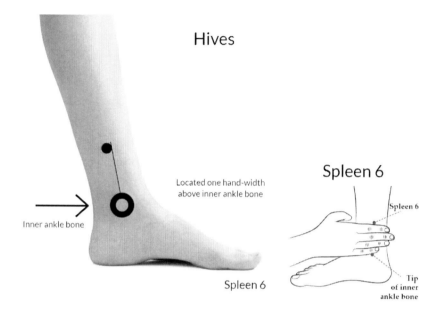

Hives

Located one hand-width above inner ankle bone

Inner ankle bone

Spleen 6

Spleen 6

Spleen 6

Tip of inner ankle bone

Treatment Notes

I treat hives with the acupuncture points and Chinese herbs that are used to treat allergies, Jade Screen and Xanthium from Golden Flower. This product is only available through licensed acupuncturists. It is great to treat allergy and sinus issues. It is based on a famous Chinese herbal formula called Jade Windscreen, or Jade Screen. The idea behind this formula is to boost the immune system and stop the allergic reaction.

Planetary Herbals has a formula called Astragalus Jade Screen. It contains extracts of astragalus root, atractylodes, and siler root. They also have a product that is astragalus root extract as a single herb. It is called Astragalus Extract, Full Spectrum.

Astragalus is a deep immune tonic. When taken regularly it will reduce allergies by boosting the strength of the immune system. In China, children are served astragalus tea. I have heard that they sometimes put the tea in food so children will not notice.

Hormonal Health

There are numerous points that improve hormone production and balance. Chinese herbs are usually combined with acupuncture for faster results. In Chinese medicine theory, aging is caused by a decline of the Kidney energy, so treating the Kidneys is a way to reduce the signs of aging.

The Kidney meridian is the first place to start for hormones. Kidney 3, 6, and 7 are the first points to use. Kidney 3 is the most important point on the channel. Kidney 7 correlates to testosterone, and Kidney 6 correlates to estrogen. That is a very basic way of looking at it, but it might make it easier to understand. Although Kidney 7 improves Kidney yang, it regulates the body and there is no downside to using it.

We all need enough hormones, and hormone balance to be healthy. Stress, aging, sleep problems, and childbirth, are a few common causes of hormonal deficiencies.

In addition to hormonal balance, the Kidney meridian also treats incontinence, asthma, and insomnia. The Kidneys are responsible for many things.

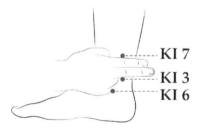

Hormonal
Health

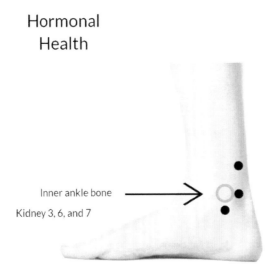

Inner ankle bone

Kidney 3, 6, and 7

Spleen 6 is one of the most important points on the body to balance female hormones. It improves hormone levels, helps your body get rid of excess fluid, relieves stress, and helps you sleep. This point is in the top 5 acupuncture points.

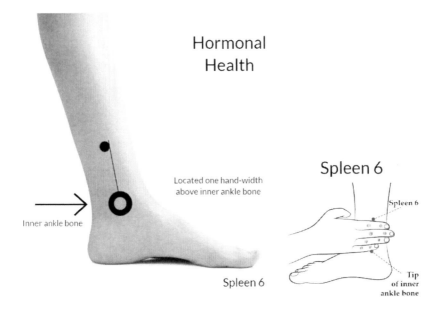

Hormonal
Health

Spleen 6

Located one hand-width
above inner ankle bone

Spleen 6

Inner ankle bone

Spleen 6

Tip
of inner
ankle bone

Liver 3 treats stress via balancing the Liver energy. It is a very calming point and most people also get acupuncture on this spot. It is one of the best points on the body to relieve stress.

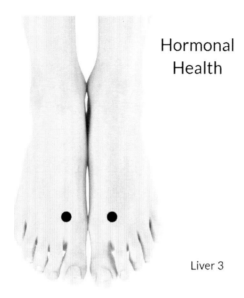

Hormonal
Health

Liver 3

Hot Flashes

In Chinese medicine theory hot flashes are usually caused by weak kidney energy. As we age, our kidney yin declines, which is responsible for many signs of aging in men and women. Although it is more noticeable in women.

Hot flashes are caused by your body responding to a lack of estrogen. There is a lot of disagreement in Western medicine about which hormone is most important in treating hot flashes and other symptoms such as vaginal dryness, insomnia, fatigue, irritability, and all of the other delights of aging. Some people say that progesterone is the most important hormone to replace. Others say estrogen is what you need to replace.

In my experience, bioidentical hormones can stop the symptoms of menopause and perimenopause, but they are not as effective as Chinese herbs in treating all aspects of hormone weakness. I believe there are hormones that have not been recognized by Western medicine. Taking bioidentical hormones can be very tricky.

The kidney meridian is the most important to treat hot flashes. Kidney 6 is for kidney yin, or estrogen. However any kidney deficiency can cause hot flashes, so I would treat the top 3 points on the kidney meridian.

Kidney 3, 6, 7. These points also treat fatigue, urinary weakness and incontinence, as well as weak bladder. I would treat these three points together.

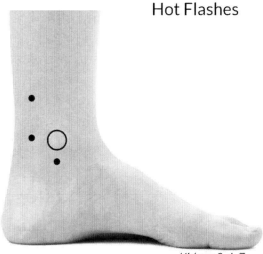

Hot Flashes

Kidney 3, 6, 7

Treatment Notes

Phytoestrogen is usually derived from yams. Solaray makes a product called phytoestrogen. This will stop hot flashes in a day or two. I prefer this over bio-identical hormones personally. Although there are many products available over the counter and I certainly believe women should get relief as quickly as possible, while they search for good long-term options.

It is not recommended to take estrogen long term without progesterone. There is always a balance in hormones, and it is possible that too much of any type of estrogen treatment might cause problems.

Chinese herbs bypass this problem. Kidney tonics can be used that help your body to make its own hormones. They also need to be monitored, as you need to balance your yin and yang, and treat digestion. Chinese herbs can restore the body back to how it was before you started losing hormones. You will notice more head hair growth, and better eyelashes.

I believe Chinese herbs restore the endocrine system much better than bioidentical hormones.

Another option that can be effective is to take herbal formulas designed for the liver. This is becoming more popular. One option is called Jia Wei Xiao Yao San, which is called Free and Easy Wanderer. Planetary Herbals makes a product called Bupleurum Calmative Compound. It contains Dang Gui, atractylodes, peony root, poria, ginger root, licorice root, mint, and bupleurum root.

This formula is based on Jia Wei Xiao Yao San, and it is one of the premiere formulas to treat stress, hormone imbalances, infertility, irritability, and many other problems.

Impotence, Libido

Libido issues in men and women are commonly caused by weak kidneys. As we age, the kidneys become weak, and hormone production declines. The kidney meridian is important to strengthen the kidneys.

Kidney 3 is the most important point on the meridian. It treats all aspects of the Kidneys in Chinese medicine. Kidney 7 is especially good to strengthen the Yang, or testosterone, and Kidney 6 is for Yin, and estrogen. There is no exact correlation between Western medicine and Chinese medicine, but that is close as I can get.

Strengthening the kidneys will also treat incontinence. Although the kidneys get weaker as we age, it is easy to treat with acupuncture and Chinese herbs.

Impotence,
Libido

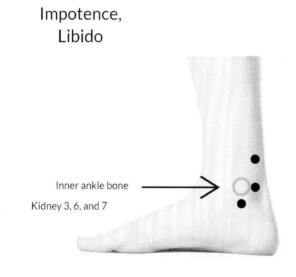

Inner ankle bone

Kidney 3, 6, and 7

Treatment Notes

Kidney tonic herbs are used for anti-aging benefits in Chinese medicine. Treating the kidneys essentially boosts the production of hormones. Aging is a function of declining hormone levels and kidney energy in Chinese medicine theory.

Horny goat weed and other herbs are popular with men. They increase testosterone naturally. I do not recommend taking herbs like this without getting advice from an acupuncturist who has training in Chinese herbs. If you take yang tonics, which increase testosterone, and you do not balance that with herbs that increase other hormones, you can easily cause a hormonal imbalance.

Taking yang tonics alone (testosterone), without the yin (estrogen), can cause insomnia, irritability, and facial hair growth in women. There is almost no way to explain how rejuvenating kidney herbs can be. They restore the body in ways that bio-identical hormones simply cannot.

We all need the drive we get from our kidneys. Weak kidneys are a common cause of depression. We simply lose our drive as we age. Taking kidney tonic herbs such as cordyceps can be an effective and balanced way to stay as healthy as possible.

Chinese herbal formulas combine the yin and yang, estrogen and testosterone. It is not good to take yang tonics like horny goat weed, which is called Yin Yang Huo in Chinese medicine, without balancing it with herbs such as Rehmannia. Herbal tonics can be taken long term to restore kidney health.

An acupuncturist friend of mine was having male performance issues, so he started taking an herbal formula daily. He no longer has issues, and his overall health is much better. This is a maintenance issue. He continues to take them to maintain his health.

When we age, our hormones decline. Taking Chinese herbs can treat all types of hormone imbalances including performance issues, hot flashes, insomnia caused by hormone decline, and many other problems.

An herbal product that is available over the counter is Cordyceps Power from Planetary Herbals. It could be too strong for some women. You don't really know how deficient someone is until you start to treat them and put them on herbal tonics. You watch for symptoms to be sure the formula is not too strong. The most common problem is when women take yang tonic herbs when they are also very deficient in yin, or estrogen. That can cause hot flashes. It is always about the balance. Everyone is different and should be monitored.

One herb that is especially helpful for libido is Goji berries. The Chinese name is Gou Qi Zi. Goji berries nourish the kidneys and liver. It is said in Chinese herbal folklore that if a man is planning to travel long distances from home, he should not eat a lot of Goji berries. They strongly boost libido in other words. Goji berries are excellent for your eyes. They are used to treat the eyes, they are said to brighten the eyes, which means that after you take them a while your eyes are healthier looking and shiny.

Goji berries can be eaten as a snack. Look for deep red berries that are not too dried out. There are different grades of berries. Dragon Herbs is a good choice. After a while, the good quality berries get stuck together in the package. This just shows they were juicy. If the berries are all dried out, they will not stick together as easily.

In my opinion, acupressure alone will not be enough to treat impotence. Chinese herbs are important and there are other possible causes of this problem, which acupuncture can also treat. See a licensed acupuncturist for help.

Infertility

Chinese medicine treats infertility by regulating and restoring hormone levels. It treats the underlying causes of infertility. There is nothing that is as effective at improving fertility as Chinese medicine.

Kidney 3, 6, 7 treat the kidneys, which treats the hormones. Kidney 3 is located behind the inner ankle bone, Kidney 7 is 2 cun above that, and Kidney 6 is located just below the inner ankle bone. Two cun is measured using the patient's two fingers.

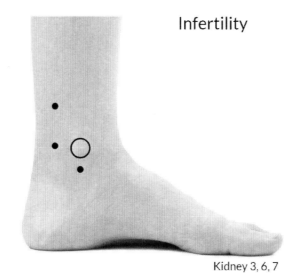

Infertility

Kidney 3, 6, 7

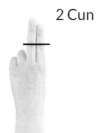

2 Cun

Spleen 6 is used to boost the kidneys which improves hormone levels. It also nourishes the blood, which means that it improves the quality of the blood, which helps to relieve many hormonal issues.

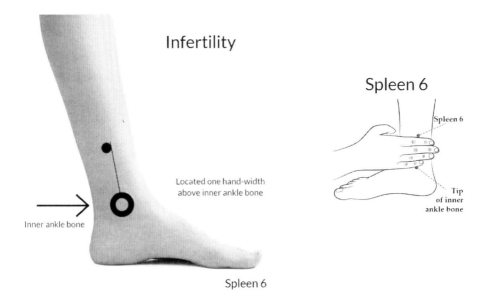

Infertility

Located one hand-width above inner ankle bone

Inner ankle bone

Spleen 6

Spleen 6

Tip of inner ankle bone

Spleen 6

Liver 3 regulates the Liver. Treating the Liver regulates hormones, relieves stress, and helps the body relax. Being stressed causes tension, so things to not work like they should. Liver 3 is located in the hollow between the first and second toes. If you rub your finger in the area between the toes, you will find a small dip.

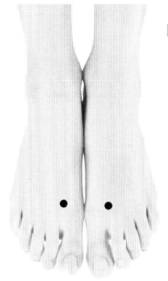

Infertility

Liver 3

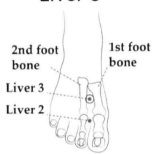

Liver 3

2nd foot bone

1st foot bone

Liver 3

Liver 2

Regardless of the underlying pattern, most people should have their kidneys strengthened, because that boosts hormone levels. There is no downside to regulating the kidneys.

There is always a cause for infertility. Even if medical doctors have told you that they cannot find a cause for your infertility, Chinese medicine can treat the root cause, which is done by using Chinese medicine diagnosis.

A point that might not be strong enough if treated solely as an acupressure point is the Uterus Point. It is located 4 cun below the belly button, and three cun from the midline, which is the line in the middle of the body at the belly button. The location correlates to the ovaries. It regulates the ovaries and uterus, but it can also regulate the fallopian tubes. I have read many case studies of people with twisted fallopian tubes who were treated with acupuncture and the tubes were restored. Acupuncture improves blood flow and restores circulation, so the body can be healthy again.

Infertility

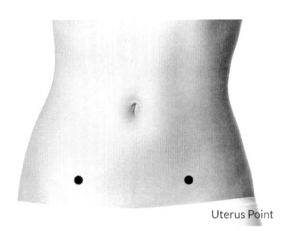

Uterus Point

Treatment Notes

Before you try Western medicine, you might consider getting acupuncture for a couple of months. The standard time recommended is three months. Many patients get pregnant before three months are over. One of my patients got pregnant after two weeks of acupuncture. Her ovulation was just right after she came in to see me. Many women are impatient and they don't want to give their body time to heal. If you can get acupuncture, Chinese herbs, and acupressure for a few months before you want to get pregnant, you will increase your chance of conception.

Male Infertility

For some reason, women often take infertility problems on themselves and feel they are somehow lacking. The man is an important part of the equation. In about 40% of cases the male is the infertile one. They can get acupuncture and herbs also. Their hormones need to be treated, and stress can also affect male fertility.

Hormone Issues and Being Female

When our hormones do not function as they should, women often feel something is horribly wrong with them. It is a natural thing to have hormonal imbalances. As we age, our hormone production declines.

If you will give acupuncture and Chinese herbs a chance, I believe most women can get pregnant without medical procedures. Some women get pregnant in a month, but most women need to commit to three months and include their partners.

It is very common that women hear acupuncture might help, and they want it to work in 30 days. That is unfortunately how our culture is. We want instant results. This stresses women out, and unfortunately makes it less likely they will get pregnant. Stress is a common cause of infertility.

If I wanted to get pregnant I would see an acupuncturist immediately and start treatment. I would also treat myself with acupressure between treatments. There is no substitute for seeing a licensed acupuncturist. Please do not waste valuable time trying to treat yourself with acupressure alone. There are many causes of infertility, and you must get a diagnosis in Chinese medicine to resolve these problems quickly.

Insomnia

Chinese medicine has been treating insomnia successfully for thousands of years. Every patient is asked about how their sleep is, regardless of why they are getting acupuncture. Insomnia can be treated at the same time as other ailments. Healthy sleep is an important part of healing.

You do not need to understand this or believe it to use acupressure to help yourself, but I wanted to give you a little information on it.

Insomnia is diagnosed via organ patterns. The heart is usually involved. Points that treat the heart are Heart 7 and Pericardium 6.

Heart 7 treats anxiety, and other heart issues. It is the number one point to treat anxiety and insomnia. It is located at the wrist, by the tendon.

Insomnia

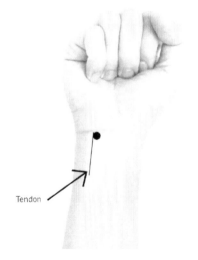

Tendon

Heart 7

Pericardium 6 also treats the heart. It also improves circulation in the heart and stomach. I sometimes send patients home with magnetic pellets to use before bed to help them get to sleep and stay asleep. These pellets are pretty strong and should not be used long term. Pericardium 6 is two cun from the wrist crease, in the middle of the wrist. I would use a mini massager on this point for five minutes at least an hour before bedtime.

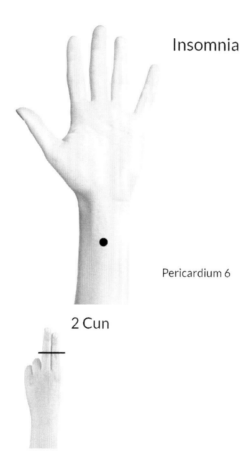

Insomnia

Pericardium 6

2 Cun

Spleen 6 helps to calm the mind, regulate the hormones, and the liver. It is a very calming point. It is one hand width, or 4 cun above the inner ankle bone, just behind the shin bone.

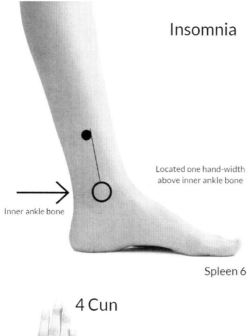

Insomnia

Located one hand-width
above inner ankle bone

Inner ankle bone

Spleen 6

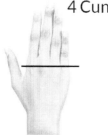

4 Cun

Kidney 6 is one of my favorite calming points. It is located below the inner ankle bone. If you have adrenal fatigue, which is caused by too much stress, Kidney 6 will help the kidneys calm down and produce the hormones you need to get to sleep and stay asleep. You should not use this point if you are pregnant.

Insomnia

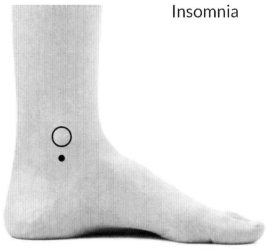

Kidney 6

Liver 3 treats stress. This point will help your body relax. Being able to relax will help you get to sleep. Stress affects your liver. This point will not only help you to relax, but you will feel more relaxed over time, as it treats the root cause.

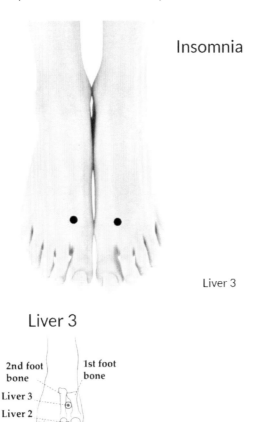

Insomnia

Liver 3

Liver 3

2nd foot bone   1st foot bone

Liver 3
Liver 2

Treatment Notes

There are so many supplements that will help you sleep. I wrote a book about this, called *Insomnia Relief*. I will include a few of my favorite sleep supplements from this book.

Flower essences are diluted extracts of flowers that treat the emotions. Bach Flower Essences Rescue Sleep includes flowers that relieve stress and anxiety. It also contains White Chestnut flower, which stops repetitive thoughts. Most of my patients feel like they have taken a sleeping pill after taking this formula, it is that relaxing. It is completely safe and does not contain drugs.

Bach Rescue Remedy formula can be used during the day to relieve stress and anxiety. They make a spray that is very convenient. Just spray it in your mouth, and also your drink.

You will be surprised how relaxed you are. Bach flower essences are preserved with alcohol, which is not a problem for most people, but alcohol-free options are available.

There are dozens of Chinese herbal formulas that treat the root cause of insomnia. If you have a serious sleep problem, please consider seeing a licensed acupuncturist. There are formulas that are taken during the day to treat the root, and formulas that can be taken in the evening to calm you down and help you sleep through the night. These herbs have been used for thousands of years to treat insomnia.

Kidney Stones

Kidney stones are usually caused by weak kidneys. Boosting the kidneys will reduce the likelihood of future attacks.

I would treat Kidney 3, 6, and 7 to strengthen the kidneys.

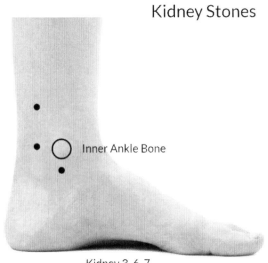

Kidney Stones

Inner Ankle Bone

Kidney 3, 6, 7

Treatment Notes

Chinese herbal formulas dissolve stones. Treating the kidneys will help you to stop making stones, but if you have already accumulated stones, you could consider herbs. Planetary Herbals makes a product called Stone Free, which treats kidney and gallstones. There are also other products that treat stones. Consider how much fluid you drink also. Your body needs water to dissolve the minerals that accumulate to form stones.

The ingredients for Stone Free are explained as "Features gravel root, parsley root and marshmallow root, historically used to promote healthy elimination of fluids from the kidneys. Includes the bitter herbs dandelion root and turmeric, to support the normal flow of bile from the gallbladder."

The name "gravel root" tells you what the herb is used for. Stones are seen as gravel. I personally like the Planetary Herbals brand because it was developed by a famous herbalist, Michael Tierra. He has written several herb books including The Way of Chinese Herbs. This book can help you to understand a bit about how herbs are used in Chinese medicine.

Knee Pain

As with all types of pain, knee pain is caused by a blockage of healthy blood flow. In order to restore healthy blood flow, you treat points on the body that restore circulation in the meridians that treat the painful area.

If you have recently had knee surgery, I do not usually treat the knee you had surgery on until the swelling is down. Treating the opposite knee is very effective and it will not aggravate swelling.

Spleen 9 and 10 are both by the knee, they open the Spleen meridian in the knee. Spleen 9 is on the inside of the leg, just below the knee. Spleen 10 is about 2 cun above the knee. Since bones are used to locate these points, I will include images from my book, *Acupuncture Points Handbook*, in addition to the flesh images made for this book.

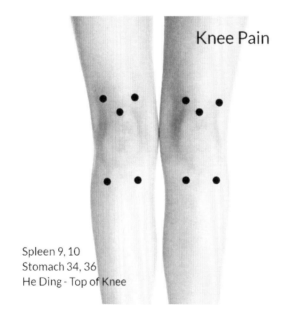

Knee Pain

Spleen 9, 10
Stomach 34, 36
He Ding - Top of Knee

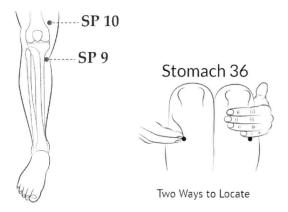

Two Ways to Locate

Stomach 34 is just above the outer knee, and Stomach 36 is located just below the knee.

He Ding is an extra point, it is not on a meridian, it is used to treat knee pain. It is located above the kneecap.

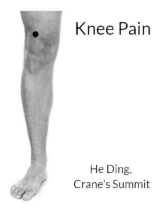

Knee Pain

He Ding,
Crane's Summit

Treatment Notes

As we age our joints wear down. Joint supplements that include glucosamine sulfate, chondroitin sulfate, and MSM can help restore joint tissue. I had recommended glucosamine sulfate for years, but found that a product that included MSM was much more effective. MSM is a form of sulfur. Our bodies needs sulfur to repair the joints. Jarrow makes an excellent product that includes all these ingredients in one pill. The dosage is 4 pills.

I have found that taking a higher dosage for a few days can sometimes speed up pain relief. This product repairs all the joints in your body, so if you have other joint problems, it will be used to repair those too. Herniated or damaged discs in the back can be repaired also. Type two collagen is also helpful to heal joints.

Lasik Dry Eyes

Lasik dry eyes is a very common side effect of Lasik surgery. Most people are not aware of this, but if you get acupuncture after surgery, you can quickly restore normal circulation in your eyes.

When eye surgery is done, the cornea is cut. When the cornea is cut, all the nerves in the cornea are cut. The nerves have to be restored for the eye to be healthy again. After surgery people often have very dry eyes. That is because the nerves that regulate the tear production are cut. Some people have chronic dry eyes after surgery.

I had Lasik myself, so before I had the surgery, I had done research and learned about dry eyes. I knew that after surgery I would be farsighted temporarily, and not able to read my acupuncture books to fix the problem. So I did my research before the surgery so I would be ready. There are dozens of acupuncture points that treat the eyes. There are points all around the eyes, and points on the hands and feet that affect the eyes. You must choose what you want to treat to get the best point to treat that particular ailment.

I did research in point location books and one point was described as being useful for "superficial visual obstruction." That made the most sense to me, since you would be getting surgery on your cornea. This point is Gallbladder 1. It is on the bone by the eye. I waited about a week after surgery. My eyes were so dry, it was miserable. I used eye drops constantly, but they provided minor relief.

I inserted Gallbladder 1 and within seconds my eyes started to water. I treated this point daily for about 5 days. My eyes healed very well. The doctor was very surprised that my eyes had healed so well, because I had been three times legally blind, and they often had to make surgical adjustments on patients who were that nearsighted. I believe that because I did acupuncture to restore normal tear production, this kept the eyes naturally moist, so they healed better than expected.

For a year after surgery, I would have sudden pain in my eyes every month or so. I knew from experience treating nerve pain that when the nerves are healing you might feel a sudden pain. Think of it is a wire that has been cut, and you are trying to restore normal electric current. It will not flow normally until it is completely healed.

I have read of quite a few people who had Lasik surgery and they had eye pain forever after that. If the nerves in the eye are cut, and they are not treated to restore normal circulation, they might hurt forever. Regardless of how long ago it was that someone had Lasik, it is certainly worthwhile to try acupuncture.

I have not used Gallbladder 1 with acupressure, but I would personally try it if I were not able to get acupuncture. The points around the eyes are very sensitive and they do not require a lot of stimulation to work. Gentle pressure should be all that is needed. The point is located on the bone. I strongly recommend finding a licensed acupuncturist to help you with this.

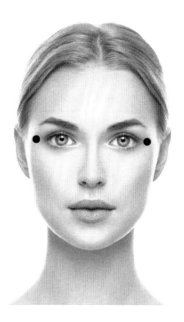

Lasik
Dry Eyes

Gallbladder 1

Treatment Notes

Seventeen years after Lasik surgery I developed horrible halos at night. The headlights on oncoming cars appeared to be a huge ball of light. It was very difficult to see at night. Someone told me that when any laser surgery on the eye is done that the proteins in the eyes are damaged. Even if you do not see the effects after surgery, over the years it can start to affect you.

I had read about some eye drops that were developed to treat cataracts. Since cataracts are caused by damaged collagen, I thought they might help me. The drops are called Bright Eyes. Life Extension foundation makes them. They contain the amino acid L-carnosine.

Carnosine helps your body to heal damaged protein, like the collagen in your eyes. I used the drops twice a day, as directed. Within a few months my eyes were 80% better. It also treated my far-sightedness that had started in the last year. As we age, the collagen does not repair itself as well on its own.

209

Many people view the eyes are being very static. They think that once the damage is done, it is like frying an egg. The damaged protein cannot be repaired. That would make sense if your eye were dead, like a fried egg. Your eye is able to heal itself if you give it what it needs.

There are acupuncturists who specialize in treating eye diseases. In addition to the commonly used acupuncture points around the eyes, there are also points on the hands and feet that are used to treat serious eye diseases. Many eye diseases are treatable with acupuncture. It works by restoring circulation to the eyes, and treating underlying imbalances that cause collagen issues.

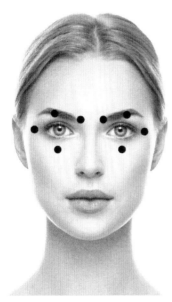

Acupuncture
Points
for
Eye Diseases

Meniere's Disease

Meniere's is classified as an inner ear disorder that can cause tinnitus, dizziness, hearing loss, and a sensation of congestion in the ear. The attacks usually come and go. Migraines are sometimes mentioned as a cause of Meniere's. I found that interesting. If migraines are correlated with Meniere's then that means that the root cause of both diseases could be the same. Migraine headaches are usually very easy to completely resolve with acupuncture, so I will give you the theory behind how it works.

Migraines are often caused by tight muscles pressing down on the nerves and blood vessels leading to the brain. In Chinese medicine, we use the channel theory. If the side of your head hurts, we treat the Gallbladder meridian, because that meridian wraps around the side of your head. I have written a book on migraines, called *Acupuncture for Migraines*. Other meridians can be blocked or restricted, which can cause migraines. We treat the affected meridians for lasting relief.

I have treated migraines many years and found that some people have simple meridian blockages that can be resolved in a few weeks, and others have complicating factors such as sinusitis, hormone deficiencies and imbalances, and stress that makes the muscles in the neck and shoulders tight. The underlying cause of the disease has to be resolved for the migraines to completely go away.

If you read the section on dizziness, you will see how easy it can be to resolve dizziness by treating the area at the base of the skull.

If I had a patient with Meniere's, I would treat it as dizziness and insert needles at the base of the skull, where the muscles insert, which is the area of Gallbladder 20. I usually treat the entire area to cover all the muscles and meridians. Be gentle in this area. This is around your spine. This area is very fragile and that is why it can easily be affected and cause a blockage of blood flow to the ear and head.

Many people have dizziness due to tight muscles in their neck. The atlas is the bone at the very top of the spine. Your head rests on it. If it is out of position, it can cause a lot of problems. This is very easy to treat with acupuncture.

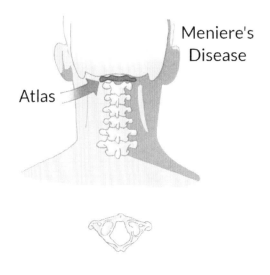

Gallbladder 20 is at the base of the skull. Since most images do not show the underlying bones and hairline at the same time, I am using the image from my point location book, *Acupuncture Points Handbook*.

Meniere's Disease

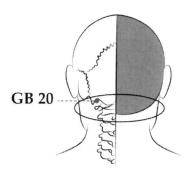

Gallbladder 20 Area

I would use gentle pressure in the area inside the circle. Since everyone's hairline is different, you need to feel around for the sore spots at the base of the skull.

If stress makes this problem worse, or makes it flare up, I would treat the Liver and put the patient on the appropriate herbal formula to treat the Liver organ pattern they are presenting. Stress makes the neck and shoulders tighten up, which could be the cause of this problem.

Liver 2 is used to treat Liver Fire, which is extreme anger and/or the face gets hot when you are mad. Liver 3 is used to treat Liver stagnation, which most people have to some degree. Treating these points relaxes the body and relieves tension on the base of the skull.

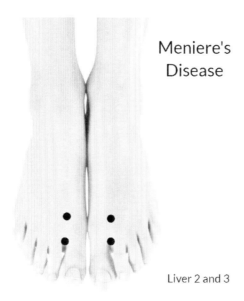

Meniere's Disease

Liver 2 and 3

If it does not make sense to you that tight neck muscles can cause migraines and Meniere's disease, imagine what would happen if you put even slight pressure on a finger, which blocked blood flow. It would very quickly start to hurt when the blood flow was reduced and the tissue did not get oxygen. It is the same with your head.

Treatment Notes

If acupressure is not enough to resolve this problem, consider acupuncture. Chinese medicine has a different system of diagnosis and treatment for internal disorders. If there is an internal imbalance causing your problem, you can get a faster resolution if you combine acupuncture, acupressure, and Chinese herbs.

Over 80% of us are magnesium deficient. This causes our muscles to be tight, because our muscles need magnesium to relax. Soft drinks have phosphoric acid in them, which must be buffered by the minerals in your body. If you drink soft drinks, I would recommend taking Raw Calcium from the Garden of Life brand. This product has calcium and magnesium, as well as other bone building cofactors. If you have drunk soft drinks a lot in your life, you probably are very mineral deficient. Raw Calcium is an organic product that has been shown to reverse osteoporosis.

Calcium needs magnesium to be absorbed. No one should take calcium as a single supplement. You should especially not take calcium carbonate, as it is not well absorbed and can cause problems. This type of calcium is very cheap, and it is often used in the products sold in discount stores.

If you prefer to take magnesium as a single supplement, magnesium glycinate is very well absorbed. The Doctor's Best brand makes a chelated magnesium glycinate product that is very well absorbed.

Migraine Headaches

If you understand how acupuncture relieves pain by restoring blood flow in the meridians, so the body can heal itself, it makes sense that acupuncture is very effective to treat migraines. Migraine headaches are like any other type of pain. There is always a cause.

Pain always has a root cause which can be treated. Pain does not spontaneously occur. Muscles tighten over time, especially when the person is under stress. These muscles press on the nerves and blood vessels, which causes pain. When you restore healthy blood flow, your body is able to heal itself.

Migraine headaches can appear on any meridian. I once had a patient who had a headache in the middle of her forehead. That was her only health problem. This was fairly unusual, because migraines are most commonly on the sides of the head. In her case, the Du meridian on the head was blocked.

I treated the meridian that restores healthy blood flow in that meridian, the Ren meridian. Within a few acupuncture treatments her migraines, which she had been treated for by numerous pain specialists, were gone.

If your migraine is in the middle of your forehead, you can treat Ren 12, 13, 14. That might be enough resolve them.

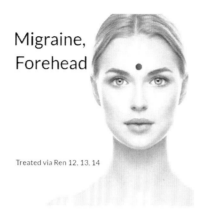

Migraine, Forehead

Treated via Ren 12, 13, 14

Migraines

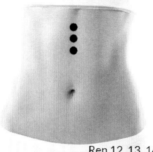

Ren 12, 13, 14

If your migraines are usually on the sides of your head, you will want to treat the Gallbladder meridian, because that meridian has a major point at the base of the skull, where the muscles attach. When that area is tight, any point on the Gallbladder meridian can hurt. You do not have to know exactly what point on the Gallbladder meridian is affected. The image below is from my point location book, *Acupuncture Points Handbook*.

If I personally had migraines I would use a mini massager at the base of my skull, at the hairline. I would treat it daily and use heat to relax the muscles there. Be gentle when treating this area, it is very sensitive. You do not need to be forceful. The body responds better to gentle stimulation.

217

Gallbladder Meridian on Head

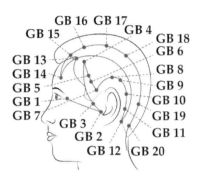

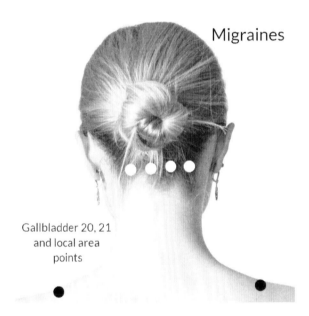

Migraines

Gallbladder 20, 21
and local area
points

Stress is the most common root cause of migraines. Liver 3 is the best point for stress. Hormone imbalances can also cause migraines, Spleen 6 is the best choice for that. Please refer to the sinus chapter to treat sinus pain. Spleen 6 is located one hand width above the tip of the inner ankle bone, behind the shin bone. Liver 3 is located in the slight dip between the first and second foot bones, between the toes.

Migraines

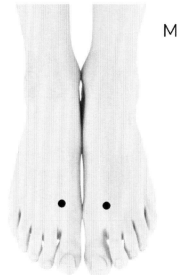

Liver 3

Migraines

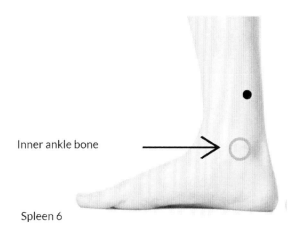

Inner ankle bone

Spleen 6

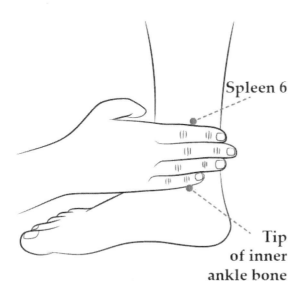

Spleen 6

Tip of inner ankle bone

Morning Sickness

In Chinese medicine theory, morning sickness is caused by a blockage in the meridians. The body has to adjust to the new baby, and the pressure it puts on the body. There are several points that treat morning sickness.

Pericardium 6, on the wrist, is the most popular point for morning sickness. Wrist bands are available that can be used throughout the day to put gentle pressure on the point.

People often do not locate Pericardium 6 correctly. It is located two fingers above the wrist crease, but you should not bend your hand back. Keep your hand and wrist straight.

Remember that each person has different measurements, so use the patient's fingers to measure the point. Men have larger hands, so adjust the measurement accordingly.

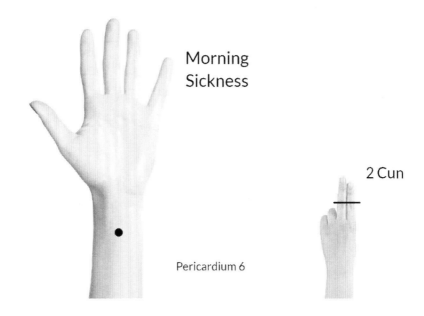

Morning
Sickness

2 Cun

Pericardium 6

If Pericardium 6 does not solve the problem, Gallbladder 34 is the next point to treat. This regulates the Liver energy, which is the most common cause of this problem. Gallbladder 34 can be a little tricky to locate. It is located by the knee, in front of and below the head of the fibula, which is the smaller bone, next to the shin bone.

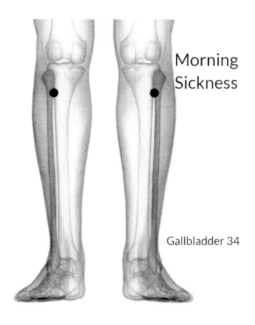

Morning Sickness

Gallbladder 34

Stomach 36 regulates and strengthens the stomach.

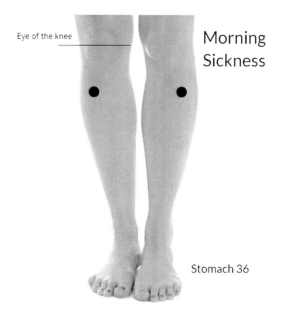

Treatment Notes

Ginger root is very helpful for nausea. It can also be used for morning sickness. You should not need to continue getting treatments for morning sickness. If these points do not work, you could try acupuncture. The stimulation is stronger and might be what you need. Always consult your treating doctor before you try anything. Every patient is different. It is best to seek the care of a licensed acupuncturist. All issues with infertility and pregnancy can be treated with Chinese medicine.

Nausea

Nausea can be caused by so many things. You would normally take the other symptoms in consideration such as if there is pain. According to WebMD, some common causes of nausea include Gallbladder disease, including gallstones, reactions to pharmaceuticals, morning sickness, food poisoning, ear problems, migraine headaches, stomach flu, ear infection, and heart attack.

The first choice to treat nausea is Pericardium 6. This point regulates the stomach area. It is commonly used for morning sickness also. If Pericardium 6 does not resolve the nausea, I would consider Stomach 36, because it is one of the strongest points on the body. It regulates the stomach and intestines.

When diagnosing health problems, it is not always easy to determine the cause of the problem. Chinese medicine is especially helpful, because we do not need a Western diagnosis. We treat the organ that is out of balance according to our diagnosis system.

The most important point to treat nausea is Pericardium 6. It regulates the Stomach. It should be the first point you try. Stomach 36 strengthens and regulates the stomach. Ren 12, 13, and 14 regulate the stomach, and treat nausea and acid reflux.

If the cause of the nausea is stress, Liver 3 can be treated. Gallstones can cause nausea. Please refer to the gallstone chapter for that information. People often underestimate how much stress they are under and how it is affecting their health. Everyone can benefit from treating Liver 3.

Nausea

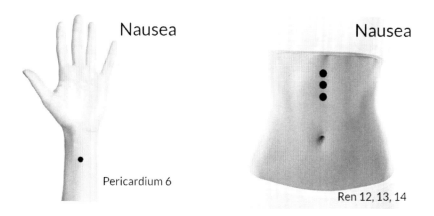

Pericardium 6

Ren 12, 13, 14

Nausea

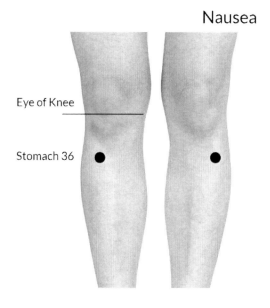

Eye of Knee

Stomach 36

Nausea

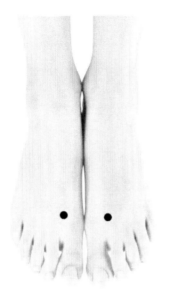

Liver 3

Neck Pain

Common causes of neck pain include car accidents, disc degeneration, neck stiffness from sleeping wrong, and holding your head in one position all day and not relaxing the muscles.

There are several ways to relax the neck muscles. My personal favorite is to use acupressure on the ears. Regardless of what other points I use on a patient, I usually place ear pellets on the area of the ear that corresponds to the neck. Every time you press on these seeds, you are improving blood flow and treating your own neck.

Treat the neck muscles directly by using a massager on the muscles next to the spine, and at the base of the skull, where the muscles attach is another good option. Warming the neck muscles is particularly helpful. Notice that these points are also used for migraines.

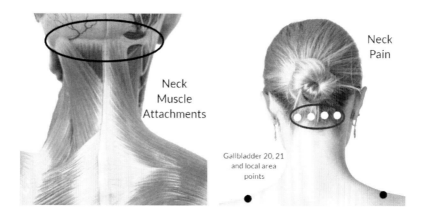

Neck
Muscle
Attachments

Neck
Pain

Gallbladder 20, 21
and local area
points

Tight neck muscles can cause many problems. When neck and shoulder muscles are tight, there is a reduction in blood flow to the head. Any problem on the head can be caused by tight neck muscles.

Gallbladder 20 is located at the base of the skull, a little above the hairline in the back of the head. Gallbladder 21 is at the top of the shoulder. When the shoulders are tight, it often affects the neck. I would massage all around the hairline, and at the top of the shoulders. Be gentle around the back of your head, it is very sensitive there.

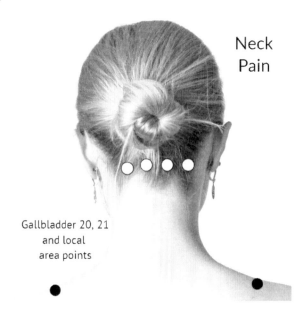

Neck
Pain

Gallbladder 20, 21
and local
area points

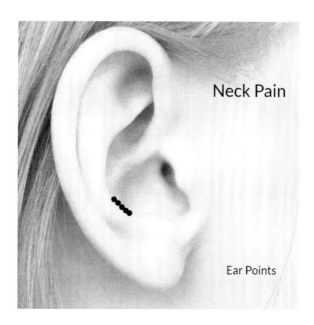

Ear points for neck pain treatment.

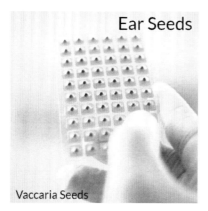

Plantar Fasciitis

Plantar fasciitis is an inflammation of the fascia, or connective tissue on the bottom of the foot. Plantar fasciitis commonly causes intense heel pain in the morning. When you sleep at night the foot relaxes. When you get up in the morning you stretch out the fascia again and it can cause excruciating pain. It feels like you just stepped on a tack.

Points on the kidney meridian restore healthy circulation in the heels and feet.

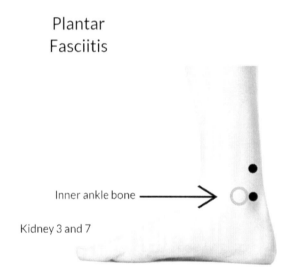

Plantar
Fasciitis

Inner ankle bone ⟶

Kidney 3 and 7

Treatment Notes
Wearing shoes with thin soles can irritate the fascia and inflame it. Wearing shoes that have no arch support can cause the arches to fall and put pressure on areas where it should not have pressure. Shoes with a good arch support are important.

There are night splints that can maintain the foot in the flexed position, which helps it to heal and relieves the pressure and pain when you first get up.

I suggest you wear shoes with a good arch support all day and night to help it heal. If the muscles and tendons in the foot are inflamed due to a lack of good arch support, providing good arch support might relieve the pain completely.

You can wear shoes all day to protect the foot while it heals. Ecco and Merrell make shoes with great arch support, and you can buy arch supports to put in your existing shoes.

Plantar Fasciitis

Pathologies Of Foot

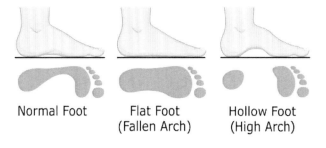

Normal Foot   Flat Foot   Hollow Foot
                (Fallen Arch)   (High Arch)

PMS

In Chinese medicine theory, premenstrual syndrome, or PMS, is caused by stagnant liver energy. Hormonal issues are often a little time consuming to resolve. A time commitment of three months is what I usually give women. There are often numerous imbalances that have to be treated. Stress causes stagnant liver energy.

Liver 3 is the first choice to regulate the liver. Spleen 6 also regulates the liver, and the kidneys. Spleen 6 treats what we call a blood deficiency, which is sometimes correlated to anemia in Western medicine, but not always. Chinese medicine can resolve problems on an energetic level, before a blood test can detect a problem.

PMS

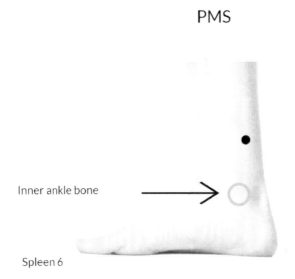

Inner ankle bone

Spleen 6

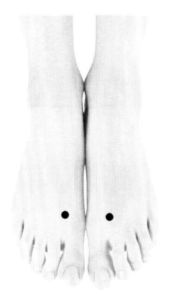

PMS

Liver 3

Treatment Notes

A Chinese herbal formula called Xiao Yao Wan is one of the most commonly used formulas to treat stress and menstrual disorders. It is also called Free and Easy Wanderer, Relaxed Wanderer, and other names that indicate it relaxes the body. Planetary Herbals makes a product called Bupleurum Calmative Compound. This formula was developed about 875 years ago. It is sold over the counter at most Chinese grocery stores. These types of herbal formulas are as commonly taken in China as aspirin is in the West.

Sciatica

Sciatica is pain that radiates down the leg. The pain can reach the foot, or stop at some point before it reaches it. This pain is often caused by lower back issues.

My favorite acupressure point for back pain and sciatica is Ling Gu, which is a Tung acupuncture point. It is located between the first and second hand bones. It is located right on the bone. When I do acupressure on this point I use a mini massager and press firmly up into the joint.

I am including a line drawing image of this point, because it is easier to locate if you can see the bones.

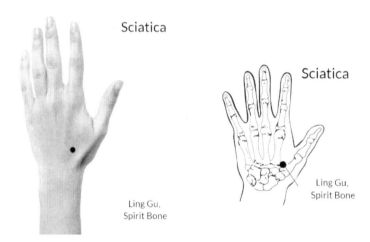

Sciatica

Ling Gu,
Spirit Bone

Sciatica

Ling Gu,
Spirit Bone

Shoulder Pain

The shoulder is very prone to chronic pain. There is a lot of connective tissue in the joint, and once it is inflamed, scar tissue can form, which causes chronic pain.

There are points around the shoulder that stimulate circulation in the shoulder and break down scar tissue. To do acupressure on these points, I would think that the mini massager would be a good option. Treat all around the front and the back of the shoulder joint.

Stretching is also helpful. When acupuncture is done, the needles break down the scar tissue. With acupressure, it might be difficult to get deep enough into the joint to access the scar tissue. Stretching helps to restore blood flow into the joint.

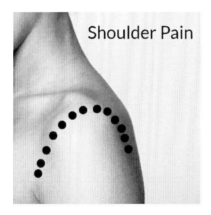

Shoulder Pain

There are three points on the hand that treat shoulder pain. Two of them are Tung acupuncture points. Large Intestine 3, Ling Gu, and Fan Hou Jue. This is a special type of acupuncture that was kept secret in the Tung family for 2,000 years. I would treat these points with a mini massager.

I would treat on the opposite side of the pain. So if your right shoulder hurts, treat the points on the left hand.

Shoulder Pain

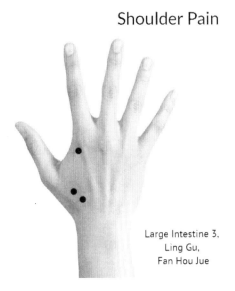

Large Intestine 3,
Ling Gu,
Fan Hou Jue

Treatment Notes

Stretching is very helpful for shoulder pain. If you get acupuncture, the needle penetrates into the joint and resolves scar tissue that can cause chronic pain and tightness. Stretching can also help to relax the tight muscles.

You can simply lie in bed and put your arm behind you. You will feel the stretch in the shoulder muscles. There is no reason to be aggressive with your stretches.

The reason the shoulder needs to be stretched so much is because of how it works. It is very sensitive to posture. It is easy to hunch over when we work at a desk all day. This can cause shoulder tightness.

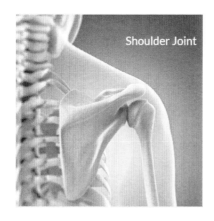

Shoulder Joint

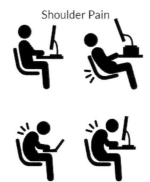

Shoulder Pain

Shoulder Stretch

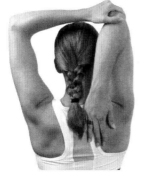

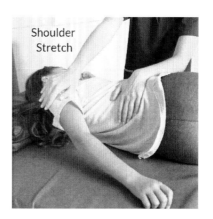

Shoulder Stretch

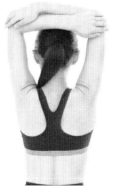

Shoulder Stretch

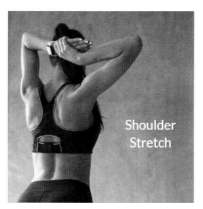

Shoulder Stretch

Sinus Pain

Sinus pain is caused by a blockage in the sinuses. When doing acupressure you might need to treat both the upper and lower sinuses, as it is hard to determine which part is blocked, if not all the sinuses.

Any headache or pain on the face, including the jaw, can be caused by blocked sinuses. There are points on the face that help to drain the sinuses, and points on the hands that treat headaches.

My first choice to treat sinus pain is the point closest to the nasal bone. I prefer acupressure on this point, rather than acupuncture, because it is very sensitive. Try all the points, because it is hard to isolate sinus problems.

Bladder 2 is at the end of the eyebrows, it can help with upper sinus problems. Jia Bi is right by the nasal bone. The point at the lower end of the nose, by the nostrils is Large Intestine 20. The image below shows Jia Bi. It is my first choice to open the sinuses and relieve pain.

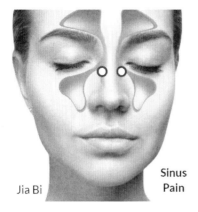

Jia Bi

Sinus
Pain

Sinus Pain

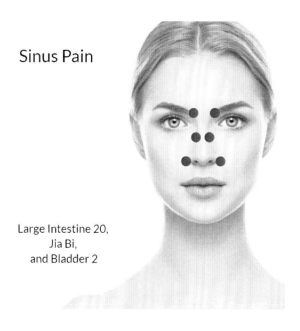

Large Intestine 20,
Jia Bi,
and Bladder 2

Large Intestine 4 can be used to treat any problem on the face.

Sinus Pain

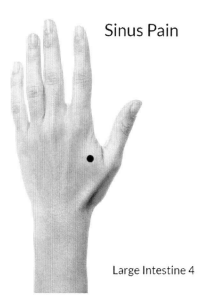

Large Intestine 4

Please note how the sinuses correspond to the acupuncture points used to treat them.

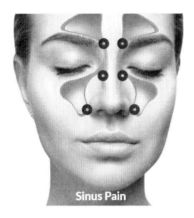

Sinus Pain

Treatment Notes

There are Chinese herbal formulas that treat allergies, sinus inflammation, and sinus infections. One of my patients had such a bad sinus blockage that he could not even smell food. Within a few months of getting treatment he had no sinus problems and could smell food again. Fungus can also grow in the sinuses. This can serve as a continual irritation to the sinuses. Immune tonic herbs like cordyceps can be used to boost the immune system to help it get rid of bacteria and fungus.

Stress and Irritability

In Chinese medicine theory, stress and irritability are related to the liver. When you experience excess stress, it affects the liver. The liver energy becomes stuck, and this causes your stress to be worse. This stuck liver energy can start in childhood. Constant criticism from a parent, or other stressful circumstances can cause tight muscles, and migraine headaches. Most of my migraine patients had their first migraines as children.

Stress builds up over time. The liver is affected and it continues to worsen over time. This is also a common cause of infertility.

The acupuncture points Liver 2 and Liver 3 are important to treat stress. Liver 3 is the most commonly used, but Liver 2 is effective for patients who suffer from Liver fire, which is an extreme form of stress. I have noticed that this is more common in patients now than 20 years ago, so I wanted to include Liver 2. It is easy to treat. You can treat both points at the same time. Liver 3 is located in the small indentation between your first and second foot bones. A mini massager would work best on this point.

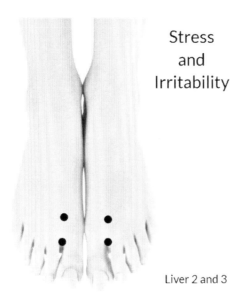

Stress
and
Irritability

Liver 2 and 3

Spleen 6 treats anxiety, insomnia, stress, infertility, hormonal issues, and fluid retention. It also balances the liver. Although Liver 2 and 3 are the most important to treat stress, Spleen 6 can also help.

Stress

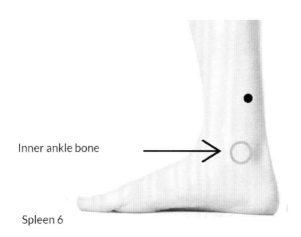

Inner ankle bone

Spleen 6

Spleen 6

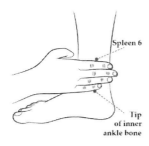

Treatment Notes

One of the most popular herbal formulas to treat liver imbalances and stress is called Free and easy wanderer, or Xiao Yao Wan. There are several variations of this formula, but the common ingredient is bupleurum. Bupleurum regulates the liver. This formula is available over the counter in Chinese markets and it is one of the most commonly used formulas. It treats the liver, and digestion. Some people are fatigued because of stress. This formula can help.

An over the counter herbal option for this is by Planetary Herbals called Bupleurum Calmative Compound. This product is based on the formula used for over 875 years to treat Liver imbalances. The ingredients are: Dong Quai Root, Bai-Zhu Atractylodes Rhizome, Chinese Peony Root, Poria Sclerotium, Ginger Root Extract, Licorice Root Extract, Chinese Mint Aerial Parts, and Bupleurum Root Extract.

Stroke Recovery

Few people are aware that getting acupuncture soon after a stroke can quickly restore normal function.

My dad had a stroke when I was in acupuncture school. It was devastating. There is always the fear that someone will not fully recover.

There are different types of acupuncture that can help people recover normal function. There is traditional Chinese medicine, which is using the body meridians to restore blood flow in the affected area. In addition to this there is scalp acupuncture, which uses needles beneath the scalp on specific points to stimulate circulation. You can also find videos on Youtube showing people recovering after a stroke when they get scalp acupuncture. There is a documentary about a man who went to China for treatment after a devastating stroke, it is called 9,000 Needles.

The main objective is to restore normal circulation in the area of the body that was affected by the stroke.

When my dad had his stroke I was in acupuncture school and only had a few days to treat him. He was concerned that I would kill him, or he would bleed out, since he was on blood thinners. I was grateful that he was treated with blood thinners to prevent another stroke, but he was limping and I knew I could help him.

His left arm was very weak, his left leg was weak and cold. I knew from acupuncture school that when part of the body is cold, it needs to be warmed up. There will be little blood flow in a limb that is cold. Heat improves blood flow.

245

He lived across the country from me, so when I saw him I did not have a lot of tools at my disposal. All I had was some moxa sticks and needles. He was not exactly the most willing patient, since he really did not believe in acupuncture at the time. In 1997, most Americans probably did not believe in acupuncture, so he was in the majority.

When treating a stroke patient, you can treat either the affected side, or the strong side. I treated both. In Chinese medicine theory, the strong side has more Qi and blood, and since the body is a bilateral system, when I treat your right arm, I am also treating your left arm. In his case, I treated the weak side, because he did not want me to treat the strong side.

I had to quickly treat him as many times a day as he would let me. I treated the strongest points on the Large Intestine meridian on the arm, which is Large Intestine 4, and 11. I also treated his hands a few times, on the points between the fingers, called Ba Xie. These points improve circulation to the hands and fingers.

On the legs I treated Stomach 36, 40, and Ba Feng, which are the points between the toes.

I applied moxibustion to the front and back of his calves. Since the muscles were cold, I was concerned that if I did not use moxa to heat the muscles, the acupuncture would not be as effective. Where there is cold, there is little blood circulation. You need circulation to heal. Cold congeals the blood in Chinese medicine theory.

In true Dad style, he took a nap as I treated him. He laid on his side and I used the moxa on the back of his cold calf. As long as his leg was cold, I kept applying the moxa heat to it.

246

I ended up squeezing his calf muscle and applying moxa for over an hour. I refused to stop the moxa treatment until his leg warmed up.

This was the most important thing I did for his leg. After the leg was warmed up he had a major turning point in his ability to walk.

A quick explanation of moxa is that moxa is the herb mugwort, or artemesia annua. It is rolled into a cigar shape and lit on one end. The lit end burns like a cigar and provides a heat source. It provides not only heat, but the herb stimulates blood flow very strongly. The rolled herb is waved over the area to be treated.

In addition to the acupuncture and moxa, he squeezed a ball in the affected hand throughout the day. This is something the hospital gave him for therapy. He worked very hard at his physical therapy to recover from his stroke. If I had been able to stay with him, his acupuncture treatments would have sped his healing.

About nine months year later I visited him again. He walked so fast I could barely keep up with him. He had completely recovered.

If he were in my office after his stroke, I would have used a TDP lamp for a heat source. I would have used the lamp to heat his leg for as long as it took to restore blood flow. Please see a licensed acupuncturist for any type of moxa therapy. Acupuncture is amazing to help with stroke recovery.

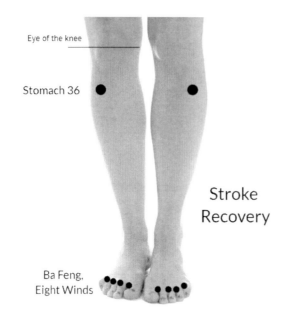

Eye of the knee

Stomach 36

Stroke
Recovery

Ba Feng,
Eight Winds

Stroke
Recovery

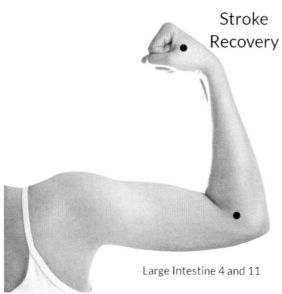

Large Intestine 4 and 11

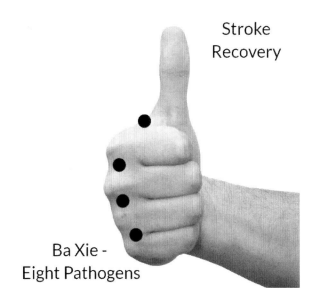

Stroke
Recovery

Ba Xie -
Eight Pathogens

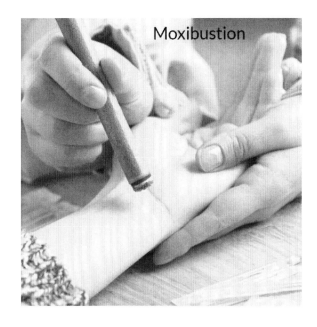

Moxibustion

Toe Pain

The points between the toes are great for any type of toe pain. These points are also used for diabetic neuropathy because they strongly improve circulation in the toes and feet. If your big toe hurts, Spleen 3 can help. It is located by the ball of the first toe.

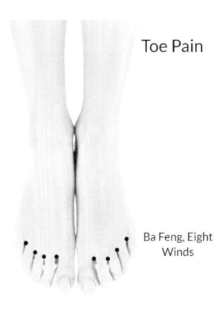

Toe Pain

Ba Feng, Eight Winds

Toe Pain

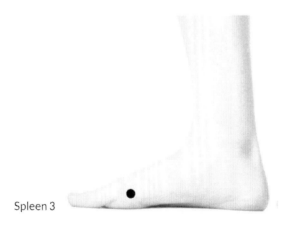

Spleen 3

Water Retention, Edema

Many people are retaining excess fluid and they don't even know it. There are two common types of edema, pitting and non-pitting. The easiest type to spot is pitting edema. Press your finger on your foot or ankle, below the ankle bone. If you press firmly for about a minute and there is an indentation left behind, you have pitting edema.

The only solution for this problem in Western medicine is to take diuretics. This does not solve the underlying cause of the problem, and they can deplete the kidneys.

The best thing to do to treat water retention is to treat the kidneys, and spleen. The kidneys are responsible for the fluid balance in your body. Strengthening the Spleen and Kidneys treats the root cause of excess fluid retention.

Kidney 3 and 7 treat the root cause of edema. Kidney 3 is located by the inner ankle bone. Kidney 7 is 2 finger widths directly above that.

2 Cun

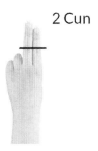

Water Retention,
Edema

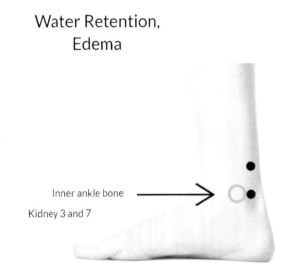

Inner ankle bone ⟶

Kidney 3 and 7

Spleen 9 is used for all types of edema. It is located just below the knee, on the inner calf.

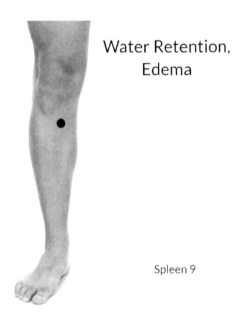

Water Retention,
Edema

Spleen 9

Spleen 6 reduces swelling and excess fluids. It is located one hand width above the inner ankle bone, behind the shin bone.

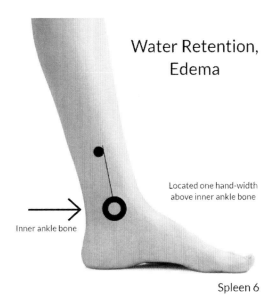

Water Retention,
Edema

Located one hand-width
above inner ankle bone

Inner ankle bone

Spleen 6

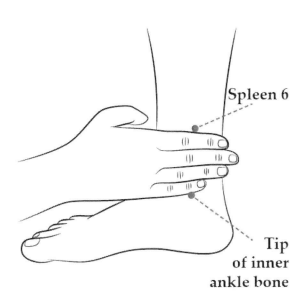

Spleen 6

Tip
of inner
ankle bone

Stomach 36 boosts digestion and energy to help your body get rid of excess fluid.

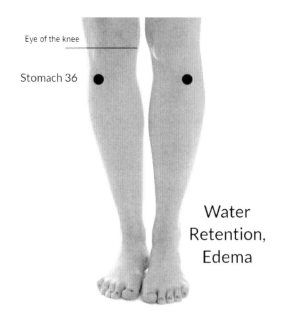

Eye of the knee

Stomach 36

Water Retention, Edema

ST 36 Location

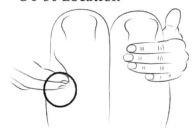

Diameter of Point

When I was in acupuncture school one of my teachers gave an intro class on acupuncture for the general public. He put one needle in a volunteer. He treated Spleen 6. This woman called the next day to make an appointment, and started getting regular acupuncture in the student clinic.

Just one needle, in one point, and her leg swelling started to go down. The needle was not even left in for the normal treatment time of 20-30 minutes.

Weight Loss

It is a common question that acupuncturists are asked. Can acupuncture help you lose weight? The answer to that is that acupuncture can help you treat problems that might cause weight gain, but it cannot overcome a bad diet.

I have had several patients who lost 10 pounds in a month. They had already been eating a pretty healthy diet, but were not able to lose weight. Acupuncture can help you lose weight in numerous ways.

Acupuncture boosts your metabolism by strengthening your kidneys, and improves digestion and elimination. It also helps to get rid of excess fluid retention. Your body must be healthy to get rid of excess fluid.

You might have heard of someone getting ear needles or seeds and losing weight. There are points on the ear that correspond to the mouth, and the stomach. Stimulating these points regulates the stomach. If you are eating too much because you have a stomach disorder, the ear points will help. They are not a lasting solution to weight loss. In addition, putting ear seeds or tacks in the ear is not effective after a few days. The points react at first, then they shut down and stop working. I use the ear to treat neck and back pain, but I alternate the points from left to right to avoid overstimulating the ear.

The points that work best to help you lose weight strengthen digestion, get rid of excess fluid, and boost the kidneys to improve metabolism.

Kidney 3 and 7 strengthen the Kidneys to boost energy levels and get rid of excess fluid.

Weight Loss

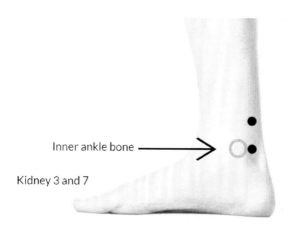

Inner ankle bone ⟶

Kidney 3 and 7

Spleen 9 is an important point to help your body get rid of excess fluid.

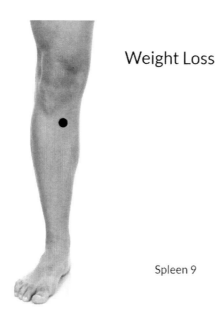

Weight Loss

Spleen 9

Spleen 6 is an important point to balance hormones, reduce swelling and fluid retention. It also treats swelling from surgery.

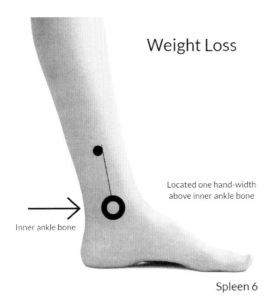

Weight Loss

Located one hand-width above inner ankle bone

Inner ankle bone

Spleen 6

Stomach 36 this is one of the most commonly used acupuncture points. It boosts the immune system, strengthens digestion, and about 100 other things.

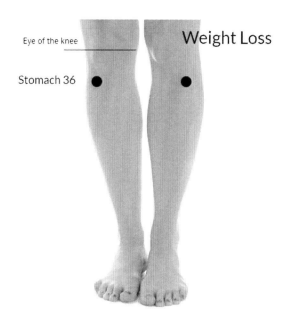

Acupuncture regulates the function of the body. It strengthens digestion, improves energy levels, and sleep.

Resources

The Foundations of Chinese Medicine by Giovanni Maciocia. This is the first year text for acupuncture students. It explains Chinese medicine diagnosis and Chinese medicine theory.

The Practice of Chinese Medicine by Giovanni Maciocia. This is the second year book for acupuncture students. Dozens of diseases are explained in Chinese medicine terms. It explains how to diagnose and treat diseases, which acupuncture points to use, and which herbal formulas to use.

Index

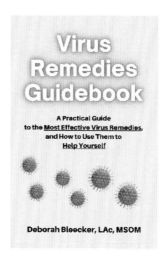

Virus Remedies Guidebook

A Practical Guide
to the <u>Most Effective Virus Remedies,</u>
and How to Use Them to
<u>Help Yourself</u>

Deborah Bleecker, LAc, MSOM

Viruses are everywhere. They cause colds and flu, and many other deadly diseases. Although most people are unaware of it, there are many herbs that have been used for hundreds of years, and have also been proven by modern science to reduce viral replication. It does not matter what type of virus it is, there are natural solutions available over the counter.

These herbal remedies are:
- Easy to use
- Easy to find
- Used for hundreds of years
- Backed by modern scientific research

This book will show you how to help yourself. You don't need to suffer, if you take the right supplements.

For details on over 400 acupuncture points, please see my other book, *Acupuncture Points Handbook*.

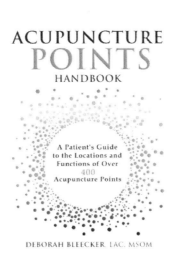

- How to locate and use over 400 points
- Easy to understand, written for the layperson
- Clear images that make the points easy to find
- Chinese medicine explained

Also, from This Publisher

Dallas Designs Notebooks, available only on Amazon. Dozens of designs. Animals, flowers, and abstract notebook designs. Three different sizes.

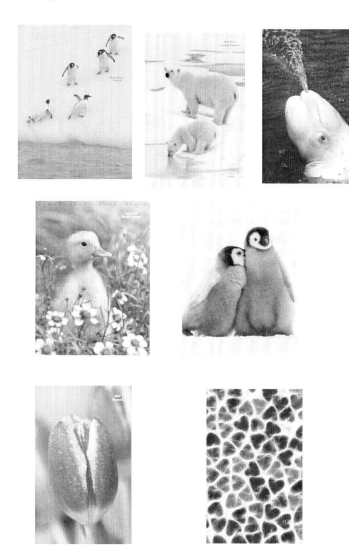

Made in United States
North Haven, CT
29 June 2023

38393992R00146